Your Weekly Weight Loss Coach

All Your Questions Answered to Drop Those Unwanted Pounds

by

Linda Owens and Kim Alp

Published by Expert Message Group, LLC

Expert Message Group, LLC
P.O. Box 949
Tulsa, OK 74101

415.523.0404

www.expertmessagegroup.com

First Printing, 2012

ISBN: 978-1-936875-07-8

Printed in the United States of America

Set in Myriad Pro 12.5/18

Disclaimer

The advice in this book is not intended for persons with chronic illnesses or conditions that may be worsened with an unsupervised nutrition and exercise plan. The recommendations are not intended to replace or conflict with advice given by a physician or other qualified health care professional. Readers are advised to seek the advice of a physician or qualified health care provider with any questions regarding personal health or medical conditions.

Contents

Introduction

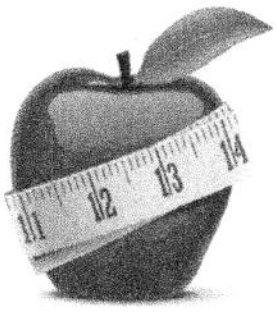

A LARGE PERCENTAGE of people who go on a "diet" to lose weight will put that weight right back on and then some. To say it bluntly, most diets are failures. Why? Diets fail because they are too confusing, too boring, and too restrictive. This book will give you simple weight loss ideas that anyone can follow. It provides basic guidelines to make your weight loss goals a reality.

With nearly two-thirds of Americans now overweight (according to the *Journal of the American Medical Association*), approximately $33 billion is being spent on diet products each year. Sadly, the only thing getting slimmer may be your wallet. This book contains 52 different strategies, one for each week of the year. It will give you common sense solutions regarding issues you deal with every day when you are trying to lose weight. You will find a multitude of approaches to weight loss that you can tailor to fit your specific lifestyle. It also focuses on *gradual* weight loss. Dietitians and physicians know that gradual weight loss is best. The pounds may come off more slowly, but they will stay off. You likely didn't gain 10 pounds in a week, so why would you think you could lose 10 pounds in a week? A one- to two-pound weight loss each week is an ideal goal. And, if you can sustain that for one year, you've just lost 52 pounds. Now *that's* an accomplishment!

Going "on" a diet implies that you can also go "off" the diet. Instead, lifestyle changes—small changes that add up over time and bring better health, more energy, and more freedom to be you—are needed. Weight loss should not be about having a Barbie doll figure, but about making a concerted effort to be healthier. Being overweight increases your risk for diabetes, high blood pressure, heart disease, sleep apnea, osteoarthritis, gall bladder disease, and complications during surgery. A modest weight loss of 10 percent will bring better health to most people. That better health may include lowering your blood pressure, lowering your cholesterol, and even the ability to control diabetes better. Who wouldn't want that?

Scientists tell us that there is no hard data to point a finger solely at one reason for weight gain and obesity. Several factors that can play a role include:

- Genetics
- The environment
- Reduced physical activity
- Large food portions
- Excessive consumption of high-calorie beverages
- An increase in the frequency of eating, partly due to an increase in readily available snack and convenience foods

While you cannot change your genes, there are plenty of these factors you *can* change. In reality, it still boils down to calories in versus calories out. We are simply eating more than we are burning.

We've all been there. You tolerate a sink full of dirty dishes, or you tolerate a car with a dusty dashboard or blackened wheels and rims. Life gets so busy that it's just easier to tolerate some things than to make plans to change them. Likewise, many people tolerate carrying around an extra 25 to 35 pounds or more. If we look at our lives realistically, the sink full of dishes or the dirty rims harm no one. But the extra 25 or more pounds keep you from experiencing a healthier and more productive life. Most people tolerate extra weight because they see the task of weight loss as daunting and unattainable. But weight loss is attainable if you take it one small step at a time.

The simple answer is to eat less and exercise more! But many people don't want to hear that, or they don't want to take a full year to do it. Besides, what foods should you eat less of and how much should you exercise? Actually, the answer is different for everyone. That's why you need to figure out a weight loss plan that suits your own lifestyle. Any weight loss plan that makes you eliminate entire food groups will only lead to failure. The key to making weight loss succeed for you and be successful for the long term is finding an approach that can be done where you live and work. The people who succeed at weight loss do not have more willpower than people who fail; they just have a better strategy.

Each strategy will provide easy-to-learn information that can assist you in your weight loss journey. If one week doesn't "match" your lifestyle, go to the next week. If you follow only five or ten of the approaches in this book and keep following them week after week, you will eventually reach your weight loss goal. This book will provide you with 52 steps to better health, more energy, and a lower weight.

WEEK 1
Small Changes Add Up

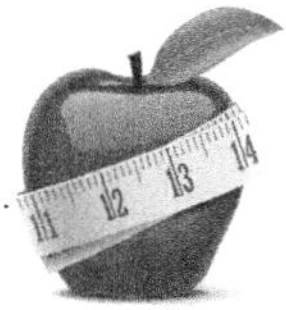

CONGRATULATIONS, YOU ARE on a journey to better health through weight loss! Remember the quote, "A journey of a thousand miles begins with a single step"? You may think your weight loss journey is like walking 1,000 miles; however, doing small things repeatedly will eventually add up.

Making drastic changes to your eating and exercise patterns usually backfires. Why? Because they are extreme and unsustainable. A steady weight loss pace of one to two pounds a week is best. This approach not only preserves muscle tissue, which burns calories better, but in one year you will have lost at least 52 pounds.

This book is about making small changes over time that add up to big benefits. The key is turning these small changes into permanent lifestyle changes, not temporary fixes. Because extreme diet regimens cannot be maintained long term, you will likely fall back into your usual eating patterns, and the weight will come right back. Also, you will likely find it overwhelming to change lots of things all at once and ultimately give up. Piecing together several small steps over time makes your goals seem more attainable.

Don't give up. It may take up to one month for you to notice results, two months for family and friends to notice, and three months for others to notice results.

Just 100 extra calories per day (1 Tbsp. of butter, 2 Tbsp. mayonnaise, 2 Tbsp. cashews, or 1/3 cup of ice cream) over 365 days translates into a 10-pound weight gain in one year. So it isn't really that we are stuffing ourselves—it's a small imbalance over time. Conversely, you can lose weight by making small changes in habits and making good food choices each day.

Look at the following suggested habit changes to help you reach your goal:

Old habit: 20 oz. cola (240 calories) and small bag of snack chips (320 calories)
Better choice: carbonated water (0 calories) and baked snack chips (200 calories)
Savings: 360 calories

—or—

Old habit: 20 oz. cola (240 calories) and small bag of snack chips (320 calories)
Better choice: a small apple (75 calories) and non-caloric drink such as unsweetened tea
Savings: 485 calories

A daily calorie deficit of about 500 calories is required to lose approximately one pound per week. So the small habit changes above coupled with some exercise will lead to significant weight loss over time.

Eating healthy foods in appropriate amounts (even if you divide them into five or six small meals) and being active (try three to four brisk, 10-minute walks most days) will give you weight loss rewards you didn't think possible. Most people who have succeeded at weight loss over time admit that it takes less effort to maintain the weight loss as time passes. It won't always be easy, but it will be worth it.

Questions to Consider

- Have I only tried restrictive, drastic weight loss plans in the past?
- Can I accomplish other goals in life (finishing a degree, completing a project) by taking one step at a time?
- Do I want my weight loss to be permanent? Do I want weight loss to occur without any effort?

WoW
Working on Weight Loss

Day 1 – Have healthy snacks on hand both at home and at work.

Day 2 – No time to exercise? Try going up and down the stairs more than necessary.

Day 3 – Do pushups against the kitchen counter while you wait for the water to boil or soup to heat.

Day 4 – Switch from refined wheat bread to 100 percent whole wheat bread for sandwiches.

Day 5 – So that you don't feel totally deprived, cut your usual evening bowl of ice cream (or other high calorie snack food) by one-third this week then by half next week. When you eliminate 150 calories per day, it translates into 15 pounds per year.

Day 6 – Divide large bags of chips or snacks into single serving sizes. Pre-portioned servings make you less tempted to eat too much.

Day 7 – Cook just enough so that you are not tempted by leftovers. If anyone is still hungry, offer them fresh fruit or veggies.

WEEK 2

Stop Starving, Start Eating

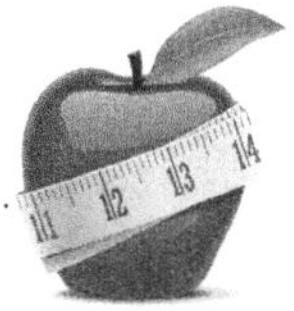

WHEN YOU STOP eating, your metabolism automatically slows down to help conserve whatever energy your body has left. When you are trying to lose weight, you want your metabolism to speed up, not slow down. When we get to Week 10, we'll talk about the importance of not skipping breakfast. But for now, it's important to know that when you eat, you actually burn calories because your body has to digest, absorb, metabolize, and store the food. Your body spends about 10 percent of your total calories on digestion alone. This is called the thermic effect of food. The more often you eat, the more often your metabolism revs up to process your food intake. Matching high fiber snacks with lean protein and healthy fats keeps your metabolism in high gear throughout the day so that you'll burn more calories.

One study found that women who ate meals and snacks at regular times throughout the day ate less overall. In addition, they burned more calories, had lower total cholesterol, lower LDL (or bad cholesterol) levels, and showed improved blood sugar.

We know that everyone's metabolism is different, just as every person is different. Once you begin to lose weight, you will not need as many calories each day to maintain the new lower weight, but don't stop eating. If you stop eating, it slows down your metabolism. Your body really thinks it is going to starve and will do everything it can to conserve energy and calories. Instead, cut your daily intake of calories by 100 to 200 and increase your exercise time or intensity.

Not eating right is one of the biggest causes of fatigue.

Never skip meals or fast to lose weight. Very little fat tissue is lost when someone fasts. Actually, our bodies lose lean body mass (muscle) when we fast. Losing lean body mass is never good because the more muscle mass you have, the higher your metabolic rate, which is what helps you burn off more calories. That's why men generally lose weight faster than women; they have more muscle mass.

Questions to Consider

- Do I routinely skip meals?
- What foods do I snack on when I eat between meals?

Day 1 – Make a list of snacks you enjoy that contain high fiber. Good examples are cereals such as bran flakes, fresh veggies, fresh fruits, whole wheat toast, or English muffins.

WoW
Working on Weight Loss

Day 2 – Set an alarm on your phone to remind you to eat.

Day 3 – Give your unhealthy snack items away.

Day 4 – Read the labels of your favorite snack foods and select the healthiest ones that contain more fiber and protein and have fewer calories. See Week 4 for guidance on reading nutrition labels.

Day 5 – Put some healthy snacks in your desk drawer or car glove box so that if times get "tough" at work or on the go, you can still eat. For instance, store some whole wheat crackers and peanut butter for a healthy snack or opt for almonds and some individually packaged applesauce.

Day 6 – Look over the hunger scale in the following chapter. If you are hungry, then eat; just opt for healthier items and watch portions.

Day 7 – If healthy, low-calorie items are unavailable, eat a very small portion of something that is not low-calorie. The main issue is to avoid not eating because that only makes your metabolism slow down.

WEEK 3

Get a Handle on Hunger

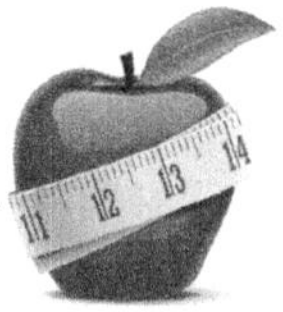

WHEN WE WERE infants and young children, most of us ate when we were hungry and stopped when we were full. However, over the years many of us have lost that ability as we were likely taught to finish everything on our plate. In addition, clever marketing has filled us with images of beautiful people laughing and enjoying themselves as they eat all kinds of food (mostly unhealthy snacks). Of course, all this plays right into our emotional need for acceptance. We know that we will never be rejected by food.

Marketing also connects us with nostalgic names like "home-style pot roast" and descriptions like "velvety devil's food cake." Studies show this type of descriptive labeling somehow makes the food taste better. Studies also show that people eat more when their attention is not directed at food. Therefore, if you eat while watching TV, answering e-mail, reading, or even driving, you actually eat more. We'll discuss this at greater length later, but for now we need to retrain our bodies to recognize hunger and fullness. It may take weeks or longer to finally get a handle on your hunger because you have likely ignored it for some time. Try rating your hunger on a scale of 1 to 10. Appendix D also lists the hunger scale.

Hunger Scale

1. You are ravenous (may be physically weak).
2. You are famished (perhaps have a headache).
3. Your stomach is empty and may "growl."
4. You are not really hungry but you could nibble.
5. You feel fairly satisfied.
6. You feel satisfied, not hungry but not full or stuffed.
7. You feel satisfied but still have room for more.
8. Now you are full.
9. You are now so full your clothes are tight.
10. You are now stuffed and may even experience reflux.

Never let yourself get to a one or two (ravenous or famished) because more than likely you will overeat in response. Most studies indicate that it takes 20 minutes for your brain to register that you've had enough to eat. Therefore, you need to eat more slowly to avoid outpacing your body's control mechanism. Stop eating when you reach a seven on the hunger scale because shortly after that you will probably be at an eight.

Most of the time people don't get very far past a four before they start eating again. This is usually because of external cues or because we don't pay attention to how hungry we are when food is readily available (at work or at home). You should try to get to a three or four before you begin to eat. Remember, you don't have to eat only three meals a day. Following your natural hunger may mean you eat five to six times a day. That's fine as long as the calories are not in excess of what your body needs.

Questions to Consider

- Am I in a hurry to eat most meals?
- Do I find myself eating because "it's time to eat" or "hey, there's some leftover cake here"?
- Am I ever truly hungry before I begin eating?

Day 1 – Study the hunger scale, make a copy of it, and look at it before you begin eating.

Day 2 – Before you eat anything, write it down on a piece of paper. The simple act of writing it will make you ask yourself if you really are hungry.

Day 3 – Make an effort to eat more slowly. Pace yourself so that your meal will last 20 minutes. See if you can be the last to finish eating. That should help you to slow down and savor every bite.

Day 4 – Keep a food journal for two days. Write down not only what you eat, but where and why you eat. You may find clues about your mood or available food that alert you to certain triggers which cause you to eat even when you are not truly hungry. (See Week 17, Keep a Food Journal.)

Day 5 – Make a list of things to do besides eat when your mood or cues say "eat," but you have not reached a three or four on your hunger scale. Some suggestions might be to return phone calls, clean off one bathroom vanity, empty all trash containers into one big bag, vacuum one room, sweep out the garage, or clean the gum wrappers, etc. from your car or truck.

Day 6 – Concentrate only on eating and enjoy every bite. Don't multitask!

Day 7 – Eat when you are truly hungry, even if it's five to six times a day, but make sure you're eating healthy foods. Fruit and yogurt make a great, healthy snack, as do high fiber fresh fruits and veggies.

WEEK 4

Making Sense of Nutrition Labels

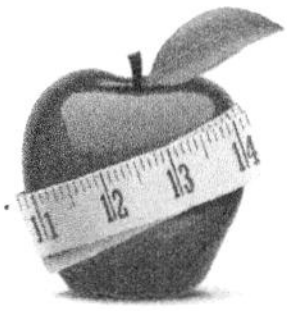

FOOD LABELS APPEAR on almost all processed foods. (A few foods that have little or no nutritional value such as coffee, tea, and spices do not need to carry nutrition labels). Labels contain an ingredient list that gives all ingredients in descending order of predominance by weight. That means there is more of the first ingredient in the product than anything else. Knowing this makes it easy to compare products.

Because labels present nutrition information "per serving," they must identify what the serving size is. Some serving sizes are set by the Food and Drug Administration (FDA). An ice cream serving size is always one-half cup and all beverages have an eight-ounce serving size. You need to compare the serving size of different products as well as compare how much you actually eat. Be careful, because some individually wrapped items such as chips, candy bars, or beverages may contain more than a single serving. The number of servings per container is listed just below the serving size.

The FDA requires that a "Nutrition Facts" panel provide nutrient information. You will see amounts for various nutrients, and they can be confusing. To begin, you may want to concentrate on calories and tackle other nutrients later. This book will discuss fat, dietary fiber, protein, and carbohydrates (starches) in other sections.

Sample label for Macaroni & Cheese

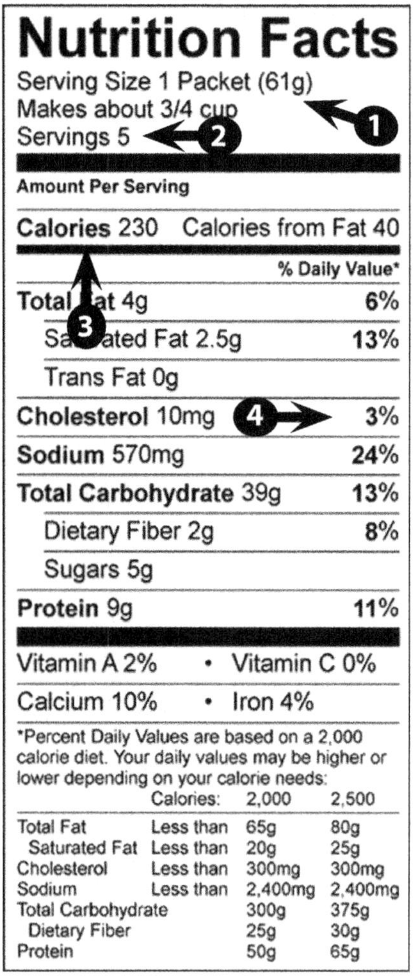

Key items to focus on when reading labels:

1. Serving Size: The portion that provides the nutrients listed on the label. You must be sure you are consuming the portion as listed or adjust nutrients accordingly.

2. Serving per Container: Don't assume that the whole container is one serving.

3. Calories per serving: Be sure you are limiting yourself to only one serving or increase the total calories if eating more than one serving.

4. Note that the **% daily values** are based on a 2,000-calorie diet.

Some manufacturers provide "health claims" on labels, but they have to petition the FDA and have scientific evidence to back up these claims. Claims that do not mention a disease or symptom require no FDA approval. Therefore, food companies can claim their product "promotes a healthy heart," "slows aging," "improves memory," or "boosts the immune system." Remember, because these claims are not backed by scientific evidence, they may be just a marketing tool, so **buyer beware**!

Today we have many items labeled "organic" (meaning it's grown or processed without pesticides or hormones) or "natural." Some of these items—especially treat or snack-type items—can still give you the same calories, sugar, and salt as their conventional counterparts. Always check labels carefully.

Questions to Consider

- Do I compare products using label information?
- Do I think reading labels is time consuming and confusing?
- Are my serving sizes the same as the label's serving size?

Day 1 – Look at the labels of three different items you consume on a regular basis. Measure or weigh the serving size and compare it to what you actually eat.

Day 2 – Look at the labels of these same three items and read the list of ingredients. Are they healthy ingredients like whole wheat flour or peach puree, or are they less healthy ones like sugar or sucrose?

Day 3 – Choose one section of items in the grocery store (perhaps cold cereal) and compare the serving sizes and calories per serving of the ones you usually eat. Decide which ones would be the healthiest.

Day 4 – Take those same grocery store items and compare the amount of protein in each serving. Remember, protein helps you feel full longer, so protein is an important part of any weight loss plan.

Day 5 – Again, take those same grocery store items and compare the amount of fiber per serving. Like protein, fiber helps you feel full longer, and it is also an important part of any weight loss plan.

Day 6 – Look at individually packaged foods you normally purchase to see if the package contains one or more servings.

Day 7 – Make a habit of looking at labels for any new food you want to purchase. Make sure it contains healthful ingredients and fits into your calorie allotment for the day.

WEEK 5

Calculate Your Calorie Goal

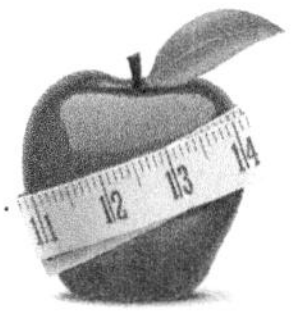

A WEIGHT LOSS of just 10 percent has been shown to provide health benefits such as lowering blood pressure and dropping cholesterol levels. Once you reach your 10 percent goal, you can set a new target weight. By doing this, you are setting realistic, achievable, and sustainable goals.

To get started, determine how many calories you need to maintain your current weight. Begin by determining your "resting energy needs." This is the number of calories your body needs at rest, such as while sleeping. The most reliable prediction equation of resting energy needs in overweight adults is the Mifflin-St. Jeor equation below. Use the following conversions to complete the equation.

Men = (10 x actual weight in kg) + (6.25 x height in cm) – (4.92 x age) + 5

Women = (10 x actual weight in kg) + (6.25 x height in cm) – (4.92 x age) – 161

Weight in kg = weight in pounds divided by 2.2
Height in cm = height in inches times 2.54

Example:

Lisa weighs 300 lb. (136 kg) and is 5'5" (165 cm) tall. She is 48 years old and has a desk job with little to no exercise.

(10 x 136) + (6.25 x 165) – (4.92 x 48) - 161 = 1,994 calories
1,994 x 1.2 activity factor = 2,393 calories/day to maintain weight

Eat 300 fewer calories daily (2,093) and burn 200 calories from exercise for a 500-calorie deficit and about a one-pound weight loss per week.

This calculation is the number of calories your body uses at rest so you will need to multiply your answer by an activity factor to get a true picture of how many calories you burn each day. See the following table and use the best figure for you.

Activity Factor	Category	Definition
1.2	Sedentary	Little or no exercise and a desk job
1.375	Lightly Active	Light exercise or sports 1-3 days a week
1.55	Moderately Active	Moderate exercise or sports 3-5 days a week
1.725	Very Active	Hard exercise or sports 6-7 days a week
1.9	Extremely Active	Hard daily exercise or sports and a physical job

After including an activity factor, the calculation will give you an estimate of how many calories you need to maintain your current weight. It takes an extra 3,500 calories to gain one pound; therefore, if you want to lose one pound each week, you need to reduce your caloric intake by 500 calories per day (3,500/7 days = 500). If you want to lose two pounds a week, you will need to subtract 1,000 calories each day. However, medical experts will tell you that your goal should not cause you to eat fewer than 1,200 calories per day. It is extremely difficult to get all essential nutrients (proteins, vitamins, and minerals) with a diet of fewer than 1,200 calories daily. Any diet that advises fewer than 1,200 calories per day should be medically supervised.

For most adult women, a goal of 400 calories per meal plus two or three 100-calorie snacks should produce good results. If you aren't much of a breakfast eater, you may want to have 300 calories at breakfast, 400 at lunch, 500 at dinner, and two or three 100-calorie snacks. For most adult men, a goal of 600 calories per meal, plus two or three 100-calorie snacks is ideal.

It will be easier to accomplish your goal if you exercise because exercise burns calories. People who combine diet and exercise typically lose more fat and have more muscle than those who only reduce calories. For example, to make up your 500-calorie daily deficit, you could reduce your food intake by 300 calories and burn 200 calories with exercise. See Week 16 for more ideas.

If you find that you are not losing weight or are losing weight too quickly (this can result in rapidly regaining your lost weight) with your calculated goal, you will need to adjust it. **Your calculated goal is only an estimate to get you started.** In order to determine if you are on the right track with your caloric goal, monitor your hunger, your energy level, your weight, and your body mass index (BMI). BMI is a useful tool that tells people if they are overweight or even if they are obese. It measures a person's weight in relation to their height, and it provides an estimate of body fat. Therefore, the higher your BMI, the higher your risk for certain diseases, such as type 2 diabetes and heart disease. You may calculate your BMI by going to a resource website such as www.nhlbisupport.com/bmi or by referencing the BMI table in Appendix B. You may also determine your current BMI by using the following equation.

To Calculate Your BMI

1. Multiply your weight (in pounds) by 703.
2. Divide the answer in Step 1 by your height (in inches).
3. Divide the answer in Step 2 by your height (in inches) to get your BMI.

Once you have calculated your BMI, you can evaluate it against the following scale to determine which category you are in:

- Underweight: BMI below 18.5
- Normal weight: 18.5 to 24.9
- Overweight: 25.0 to 29.9
- Obese: 30.0 and above

**While BMI is accurate for most people, it may overestimate body fat in people who are very muscular and may underestimate body fat in people who have lost muscle.*

Questions to Consider

- Are you aware of how many calories you consume daily?
- Do you know approximately how many calories you burn daily?

Day 1 – Set a realistic weight loss goal and write it down so that you can post it in a prominent area you'll see each day.

Day 2 – Estimate your current caloric needs and subtract 500 calories for weight loss. Then begin recording what you eat daily and compare that to your caloric needs.

Day 3 – Purchase a pedometer or use the pedometer on your iPod or smart phone to measure your steps each day. Beginners should take at least 2,000 steps per day.

Day 4 – Make a positive statement today: "I can achieve my weight loss goal!"

Day 5 – Ask your family and friends to help you with your weight loss plan by periodically checking with you regarding your progress.

Day 6 – Weigh first thing this morning and mark it on a chart. Weigh again in seven days.

Day 7 – Look at the BMI table and determine what your weight will need to be in order to have a healthy BMI.

WEEK 6

Balance Your Meals

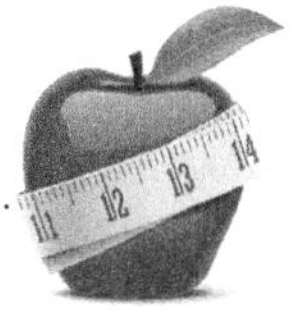

WEIGHT MANAGEMENT IS really just energy balance. It is simply a balance of calories eaten and calories burned by activity or exercise. Healthy weight management also requires a balance in the foods you eat. Do not eliminate or severely restrict any one food group, such as carbohydrates (or starches). Carbohydrates are the body's preferred energy source. Rather than follow a low-carbohydrate diet, you need to be selective about your carbohydrate sources. Limit carbohydrates that have no nutrients but lots of sugar, such as regular soft drinks, candies, and desserts. Continue to eat complex carbohydrates such as whole grains (look for whole grain breads, cereals, and pastas), fruits, and vegetables. Be sure to include low-fat protein foods such as lean meats, fish, chicken, nuts, beans, and low fat dairy. These sources of protein keep you feeling full longer.

Eat a variety of foods to obtain adequate amounts of protein, carbohydrates, vitamins, and minerals. The more colors on your plate, the healthier it is likely to be. The old method of centering a meal around meat and starch is no longer necessary or even desirable. In order to help ensure you are eating a healthy variety, begin with a nine-inch plate. Fill one-quarter of your plate with whole grain foods and fill one-quarter with protein foods such as lean meats, poultry, fish, or tofu. The remaining half of your plate should be filled with non-starchy vegetables or fruits, such as cooked carrots, broccoli, asparagus, grapes, sliced apples, or strawberries.

Design a Healthy Plate

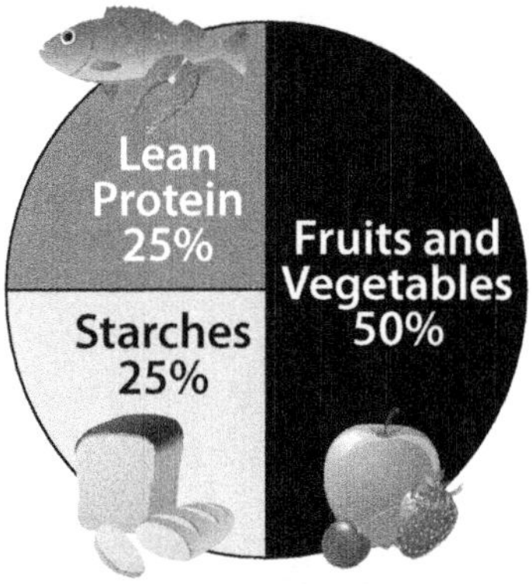

Try to eat meals at about the same time each day. Starting your day with a healthy breakfast is always best. Week 10 discusses the metabolic jump-start a good breakfast gives you. It also gets you on track with regular meals and snacks throughout the day. Be sure to plan ahead for meals, while still paying attention to your hunger scale.

Questions to consider:

- How colorful is the meal on my dinner plate?
- Have I eliminated any one group of foods?
- Do I concentrate on which meat to serve and forget about nutrient-rich fruits and vegetables?

Day 1 – Start your day with a healthy breakfast.

Day 2 – Try a new fruit or vegetable today, like mangos or beets.

Day 3 – Make sure juices are 100 percent pure fruit juice.

Day 4 – Limit sugary drinks or energy drinks to one daily.

Day 5 – Fill half your plate with veggies or salad greens, one quarter with lean protein (grilled or roasted meat, fish, or poultry) and one-quarter with a starchy carbohydrate (brown rice, baked potato, whole wheat pasta).

Day 6 – Check the label on your bread. Is it made with 100 percent whole wheat flour? How much fiber per serving does it contain?

Day 7 – Do not eat a meal or snack until your hunger scale is at a three or four.

WEEK 7

Portion Distortion

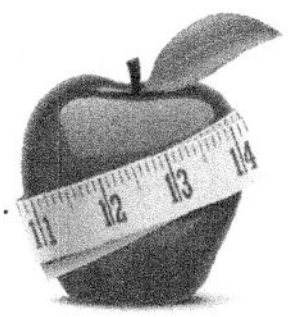

EVEN THOUGH LOW-CALORIE and low-fat foods have fewer calories, you cannot eat unlimited quantities. Everyone needs a certain number of calories each day to fuel his or her body, but when we get more than we need, our bodies store it as fat. Fat storage is a very efficient process. Therefore, when you exceed your caloric needs you will gain weight even if you are eating nutritious foods.

To avoid this situation, we should all be watching portion sizes. Just because a 12-ounce T-bone steak fits on your plate doesn't make it a single serving. To make matters worse, in many cases, portion sizes have drastically increased over the years. For example, 20 years ago a bagel was three inches in diameter and had about 140 calories; now, a standard plain bagel is up to six inches in diameter and has around 350 calories. Study after study shows that when people are given more food, they eat more.

At first it may help some people to weigh or measure food portions; but if that is too troublesome, try visualizing your portions. Follow these simple examples:

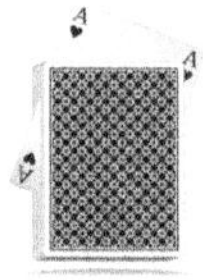

3 oz. of cooked meat, chicken, or fish is the size of a deck of cards.

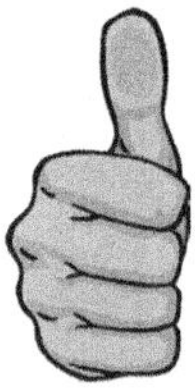

1 oz. of cheese is about the size of your thumb.

1 Tbsp. = depth of tip of thumb.

1 tsp. = a postage stamp.

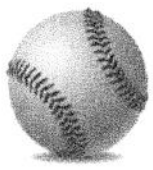

1 cup = about the size of your fist or a baseball.

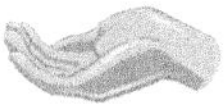

1-2 oz. of pretzels is about the size of your cupped hand.

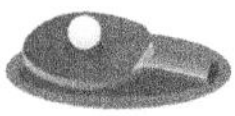

2 Tbsp. of peanut butter is about the size of a ping-pong ball.

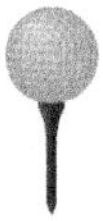

¼ cup of nuts = golf ball.

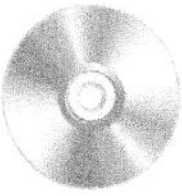

1 pancake is about the size of a DVD.

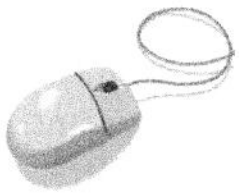

baked potato is about the size of a standard computer mouse.

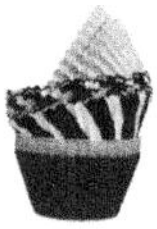

½ cup fresh fruit is about the size of a cupcake wrapper.

Once you've visualized portion sizes, there are some other tricks to help you. When it is meal time, you can place food on plates in the kitchen to avoid serving platters that could tempt you later in the meal. Ask yourself if you are truly hungry before going back for seconds (see the Hunger Scale in Week 3), or you could go against your mother's advice and always leave something on your plate.

To make smaller portions seem bigger, downsize your dinnerware. Eat from luncheon plates rather than large, 12-inch dinner plates. Studies show that when you see a bigger portion, you automatically feel fuller as you consume it, so choose foods low in calories but high in volume. Veggies and fruits are good examples.

Questions to Consider:

- Do I always clean my plate even though I'm full?
- Do I continue to nibble at leftovers when cleaning up the kitchen?
- Do I load up my plate with favorite foods rather than considering portion sizes or nutritional value?

Day 1 – Make a list of foods that are high in volume and low in calories to incorporate into meals or snacks this week. Some examples include any fresh veggies (broccoli, carrots, celery, and cauliflower), fresh apples, oranges, lettuce, popcorn, or shredded wheat cereal (not frosted).

Day 2 – Today, measure or weigh all foods before eating them.

Day 3 – Eat your food slowly and ask yourself if you are truly full before you go back for seconds. (See Week 3, Get a Handle on Hunger.)

Day 4 – Because restaurant portions are usually oversized, ask for the to-go box at the beginning of the meal. Place half your order in it so that you won't be tempted to eat the whole thing, or perhaps you could share a meal with someone.

Day 5 – Leave some food on your plate for each meal today.

Day 6 – Freeze leftovers immediately so that you won't be tempted later on.

Day 7 – Put everything on one plate so that you can see how much you're eating and *only* eat from the plate.

WEEK 8

Weight Loss Is a Process

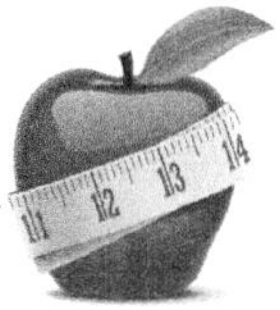

CHANGE ISN'T AN event, it's a process. Likewise, weight loss is a process. As Americans, we have gotten used to ***instant.*** We even have trouble when our computers take more than two seconds to flip screens. Slow down a little! Rome wasn't built in a day, and your weight loss goal won't be achieved in one or two weeks either. We will talk about this issue often in other chapters, but it's important to remember that any program that promises instant weight loss is too good to be true. Rapid weight loss usually means rapidly regaining the lost weight.

We need to make changes in our environment to support our weight loss journey. Without support, you'll be tempted to say, "This is too hard, so why try anymore?" Part of that support should include automating your daily life. By having the same routine each day, you'll be more likely to stay on track with your weight loss goals. Check out the WOW suggestions in each chapter to tweak your surroundings and make the process easier.

Traveling? Pack sugar-free hot cocoa. It's better than raiding the hotel room refrigerator or hall vending & gives you something sweet, smooth, and filling.

Remember, if you change your eating and activity habits gradually over time, you are more likely to stick with them and maintain your weight loss. A steady weight loss of one to two pounds a week is best because it will preserve muscle tissue. With exercise, you could even increase your amount of muscle tissue. If this happens, your weight may actually increase because muscle tissue is denser than fat tissue. Don't worry, the more muscle tissue you have, the higher your metabolism and the more calories you will burn each day. However, if you are exercising and not seeing weight loss, don't quickly assume it is due to an increase in muscle. It can take about one month to see any measureable change in muscle mass. If you are not losing weight but your clothing fits better, it is likely that you are losing fat and gaining muscle.

Questions to Consider:

- Do my past diets promise rapid weight loss?
- Have I always regained my weight and maybe more after other diets?
- Can I make my expectations fit a "process" of weight loss rather than an "instant" result?

WoW
Working on Weight Loss

Day 1 – Make a sign that says, "My weight loss is a process, not instantaneous." Read it every day.

Day 2 – Eat breakfast today and every day. Make sure on most days that breakfast is a healthy one.

Day 3 – Step back and see what progress you've made thus far. Are you eating only when hungry, eating smaller portions, or feeling more physically fit? Keep the process going.

Day 4 – Ask the waiter not to bring the bread basket to your table. Avoiding a dinner roll or slice of bread before the meal will save you about 100 extra calories.

Day 5 – If a piece of chicken or pizza looks greasy, dab it with a napkin to take off the extra fat and calories. It will save you 50 calories or more.

Day 6 – Wear form-fitting clothing or a tight belt. They will make you think twice about overeating.

Day 7 – Hang a "goal outfit" or swimsuit where you can see it frequently to remind yourself that you are working hard and making progress.

WEEK 9
Eating Behaviors

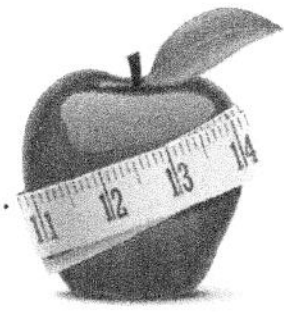

IF YOU HAVE a problem you want to solve, you first must identify what is causing the problem. As with any problem, you need to identify behaviors that need to be changed to bring about the desired result. Keeping a record of where, when, and what you eat—including what your eating "triggers" are—is a good first step. This record should help you recognize behaviors that are undermining your progress. Then you need to develop strategies that will bring about the desired behaviors and eliminate the unwanted ones. Some people call this "behavior modification." You should start small and not try to change a large number of behaviors all at once. When the new behavior becomes routine, you should move to another small change. Remember—small changes over time add up to bigger and bigger benefits.

Some areas that deserve a closer look include the atmosphere where you eat, the accessibility of food, mindless eating, and portion sizes of food and/or serving containers. The atmosphere that surrounds you when you eat plays a role in how much you eat. When an atmosphere abounds with enjoyable sounds, décor, and pleasant aromas, you will likely spend more time eating and therefore eat more. The best way to avoid this is to remove food from the table and enjoy the surroundings without visual stimulation that entices you to continue eating.

Food accessibility is also a very strong influence. Generally speaking, the more easily food can be obtained, the more we will eat. In today's world, food is highly accessible. In most towns, fast food restaurants can be found at every intersection, and every shopping center has a food court or at least several different eateries. Many studies have demonstrated that having food visible and close at hand encourages eating. In order to avoid this scenario, keep food out of sight or in an inconvenient place. In order to simplify matters, don't purchase it in the first place.

Heat canned or frozen vegetables in the microwave for a quick side dish.

Mindless eating can happen in a number of situations. It could happen when you're at a social event where food is available, and over the course of the evening, you continue to "graze" on the buffet items. It may be that you begin eating when your favorite program comes on TV and continue until it's over, or you eat popcorn at the movies even though you're not hungry. You aren't even really conscious that you are eating, but you are packing on the pounds.

There is no hope for successful weight loss until you control portion sizes. Recent decades have seen the portion sizes of foods from restaurants and grocery stores increase dramatically. Years ago, a cookie was one-and-a-half inches in diameter and provided 55 calories. Today the average cookie is three-and-a-half inches in diameter and provides 275 calories. That's a difference of 220 calories! Combine this problem with our tendency to clean our plates or finish off an entire package of chips, and we walk right into an overeating situation.

Questions to Consider

- Can I catch myself participating in mindless eating?
- What size glasses and dishes do I use?

Day 1 – Use small dinner plates or luncheon plates. Your appropriate portions will appear larger.

Day 2 – Eat foods that require a knife, fork, or spoon so that you will eat more slowly.

Day 3 – Avoid finger foods that can be consumed quickly before you realize you are full.

Day 4 – Clear leftovers from the table, wrap them, and place them in the refrigerator immediately after eating.

Day 5 – When eating out, split an entrée with a friend.

Day 6 – Always eat at a table with plate and silverware. Don't eat in front of a TV or your computer.

Day 7 – Use tall, narrow glasses for beverages. It will look like you are drinking more.

WEEK 10

Enjoy Breakfast Every Day

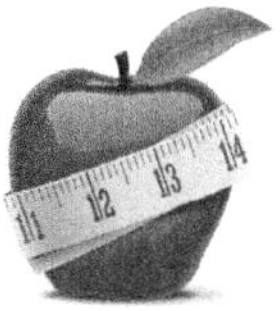

AS YOUR MOTHER probably told you, breakfast is the most important meal of the day. And it's true. But why? Research indicates that people who eat breakfast tend to consume fewer total calories throughout the day and have better cholesterol levels and insulin sensitivity than people who skip breakfast. In addition, eating breakfast gets your metabolism humming, which is what burns calories. The word breakfast literally means "break your fast" and fasting actually slows your metabolism—which is the last thing you want to do.

Studies show that a combination breakfast consisting of high fiber, protein, and complex carbohydrates or starches works best to keep you feeling full longer. Another advantage is that it helps keep your blood sugar levels more stable. In order to translate this suggestion into foods, make the following choices:

High fiber – can make a small meal seem bigger and keep you feeling full longer. High-fiber breakfast foods include whole grain cereals, breads, muffins, pancakes, and fruit. Make sure the ingredient list shows 100 percent whole wheat or oat bran at the top. Muffins can be very high in fat and sugar. (One large muffin can contain as many as 500 calories and 15 grams of fat.) Again, look for ones that list 100 percent whole wheat or oat bran first and are no bigger than three inches in diameter. Whole fruits contain not only fiber but also vitamins, minerals, and antioxidants that are good for you. Juices (100 percent fruit juice) do not provide much fiber but are still good sources of vitamins and antioxidants.

Protein – can help you feel full longer and help prevent sharp increases and decreases in blood sugar. Eggs are an excellent choice because they are not only high in protein but also low in saturated fat and calories. One study showed that when people on low-calorie diets ate scrambled eggs with toast and jam for breakfast, they lost 65 percent more weight than the dieters who ate a bagel and cream cheese. Unless you have high cholesterol, you can safely eat up to four eggs per week, according to the American Heart Association. Milk and milk products such as yogurt and cheese are great ways to add protein to your breakfast, and they also provide an excellent source of calcium—plus the low-fat versions are low in calories. Watch out for some common proteins though—breakfast meats can be laden with fat. The healthiest choices are made from turkey or soy.

Meal replacement bars are OK at times. Find one that provides at least 5 grams of protein & some fiber.

Complex carbohydrates – are foods listed under high fiber. It is worth remembering that doughnuts, pastries, and some prepackaged breakfast bars are filled with sugar and fat; therefore, they are not considered complex carbohydrates. Pancakes and waffles made with whole wheat flour are good. To make them an even better choice, skip the syrup and butter and try toppings of fresh fruit and low fat yogurt.

Be sure you are paying attention to your old eating habits and be willing to make changes like the following:

Old breakfast habit: one glazed doughnut with a 16-ounce white chocolate mocha made with 2% milk (240 + 400 calories = 640 calories)
Better choice: one bowl of oatmeal, ½ cup blueberries, and a 12 oz. skinny latte made with nonfat milk (150 + 42+ 90 calories = 282 calories)
Savings: 358 calories

Try some additional new breakfast ideas such as:

- Dip fruit into yogurt and add some peanuts or almonds.
- Blend pureed fruit or veggies into pancake batter (kids will like the different colors).
- Top a whole wheat English muffin with pizza or spaghetti sauce, Canadian bacon, and shredded mozzarella cheese, then add a thin slice of tomato and toast under the broiler for a quick, warm breakfast.

- Spread a whole wheat pita with scrambled eggs and shredded mozzarella cheese and brown in toaster oven or under the broiler.
- Make a fruit smoothie by blending a ½ cup frozen fruit, one banana, 1/3 cup orange juice, and 1 Tbsp. honey, or use 8 oz. of plain yogurt and ½ cup frozen fruit.

Questions to Consider:

- Do I skip breakfast because I'm rushed each morning?
- Do I eat lean proteins with breakfast?
- Is my breakfast healthy or laden with fat and calories?

Day 1 – Determine to have breakfast each day, even if it means eating at your work desk, but remember to focus on eating.

Day 2 – Set the breakfast table before going to bed.

Day 3 – Continue to set up for breakfast the night before—put cereal bowls on the table, cut up fresh fruit, pour and set juice in the refrigerator.

Day 4 – Hard cook eggs in advance. Then have them with a slice of whole wheat toast and either fat free milk or 100 percent juice.

Day 5 – Spread two tablespoons of peanut butter on a tortilla and wrap it around a banana for a quick, easy, to-go breakfast.

Day 6 – Stir peanut butter into a bowl of oatmeal and add a little jam instead of sugar.

Day 7 – Make a waffle sandwich with frozen, whole wheat waffles by spreading them with peanut butter and slices of banana or apples. You could also try ham or Canadian bacon between whole wheat waffles.

WEEK 11
Trigger Foods Can Trap You

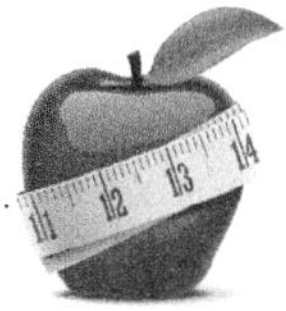

WE ALL HAVE them. Some people find that certain foods seem to trigger their need to munch, and, once they get started, they can't stop. For others, it could be the time of day or specific occasions that signal "eat, eat, eat." Whatever the reason, we need to figure out what our food triggers are and set up tactics to deal with them successfully.

One rule of human nature is that we'll never change what we will tolerate. It's surprising how much we actually will tolerate. As time goes by, we learn to "function in our dysfunction." One interesting study gave college students glasses that made everything they saw through them appear to be upside down. At first, they were lost and had to have classmates lead them around campus, take notes in class, and even help them eat. But within only a matter of days, they were walking with no problem and were even able to read textbooks and take notes. This is a classic example of learning to function in our dysfunction. Decide today to identify your trigger situations. Then determine to take control and not let them get the best of you.

How can you resist when cravings hit? First, you must recognize that your craving is like a wave. The wave rises to a peak and then dissipates. This is what happens to your cravings whether you give in to them or not. Most people think that the urge to eat chocolate will only get stronger and stronger unless they give in to it. However, giving in to the urge only reinforces it. Actually, if you resist the urge, you reinforce that resistance. Again, identify your trigger foods or situations and ride them out rather than letting them wipe you out.

Increase your fiber and nutrients by adding grated, shredded, or chopped vegetables such as zucchini, spinach, or carrots to lasagna, casseroles, and pasta sauce.

Questions to Consider:

- Can I say "NO" to that cookie that is calling my name?
- Are there specific times of the day besides meal times that I always want to eat?
- Do I have trouble limiting my intake of some specific foods?

Day 1 – Be mindful of food triggers today. Write them down as you identify each one.

Day 2 – Eliminate at least one trigger food from your pantry.

Day 3 – List one activity that you can do in order to "ride out" the urge to eat. Perhaps you could gather all old newspapers and magazines for recycling or donation, clean your makeup brushes, or organize your purse or briefcase. See Appendix E for a list of other suggestions.

Day 4 – Identify one or two situations that promote eating for the wrong reasons. It could be things like boredom or frustration or loneliness.

Day 5 – If you find yourself stressed today, exercise or meditate—don't eat.

Day 6 – Once you have identified a trigger food, look for a good substitute that won't get you off the path to good health. For instance, rather than eating regular potato chips, try individually packaged baked chips.

Day 7 – Find another path through the office that won't send you past the break room where there are cookies, candies, or vending machines.

WEEK 12

Find the Fat to Fend off Calories

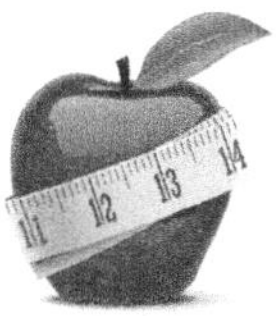

FOODS ARE WHAT our bodies use to give us energy to talk, walk, think, see, feel, etc. Our bodily functions rely on the energy we get from food. When we get more fuel than our bodies need, our bodies store it for future use in the form of fat. Calories are the measure of energy your body gets from food. Carbohydrates (starches and sugars), proteins, and fats all give us calories. Fat has twice as many calories as carbohydrates or protein. It's usually easier to cut down on your fat intake to lose weight because *you decrease your overall calorie intake twice as fast*. However, you should never totally cut fat from your diet. In order to function properly, our bodies need what are called essential fatty acids that come only from fat.

How can you tell which foods are higher in fat? Some foods are easy to identify, such as anything that is deep-fat fried, or anything made with lots of butter, margarine, or oils (e.g. pie crusts, salad dressings, or gravies). But many foods have hidden fats. Use the **Napkin Test** to identify some of these. Place the food on a paper napkin and wait several minutes. Then remove the food and check for grease spots on the napkin. Grease spots are a telltale sign that fat is present.

Pick thin crust pizza with veggies not deep dish with pepperoni and you'll save 70 calories per slice.

If you place a butter cracker and a saltine cracker on napkins, the butter cracker will leave grease spots but the saltine won't. The same holds true for a biscuit versus a plain dinner roll. Reading labels would give you the same information without the napkin (see Week 4). Some people will make healthy food choices like a grilled chicken salad and then add high-fat salad dressing. (Just two tablespoons of regular dressing provides 110 calories.) Oops, that healthy salad just turned into a high-fat and high-calorie salad!

All fats are high in calories; however, science tells us that some fats are healthier than others. Omega-3 fatty acids are proven to be beneficial to health. One of the omega-3 fats is found in flaxseeds, walnuts, and their oils. Canola and olive oils also contain omega-3 fats. Other sources of omega-3 fats include fish such as herring, salmon, sardines, oysters, trout, and tuna. Dietitians and physicians recommend that 25 to 30 percent of your total calories come from fat. If your daily caloric intake is 1,800 calories, then 450 to 540 calories can come from fat (or 50 to 60 grams of fat). Your fat intake should include the good fats listed above. Other fats called saturated fats have been shown to increase the risk of heart disease and some cancers. Sources of saturated fats include animal fats like bacon, lard, or butter, as well as coconut and palm oils. No more than 10 percent of your fat intake should come from these foods.

Questions to Consider:

- Are my food choices lean or greasy? (Hint: *crispy* and *crunchy* usually means the food is fried.)
- Is there always fat-laden salad dressing at the bottom of my salad?
- Would the foods I usually eat pass the napkin test? If they wouldn't, which foods can I use as a substitution?

Day 1 – Avoid all fried foods for three days.

Day 2 – Steer clear of any food on the restaurant menu that says *crispy* or *crunchy*.

Day 3 – Skip the cheese and bacon on your burger and pile on the lettuce, tomato, and onion.

Day 4 – Trim all visible fat from meat before cooking.

Day 5 – Cook (bake, broil, roast) poultry without the skin. (Poultry skin is high in fat.)

Day 6 – Don't pour high-fat salad dressing on your salad. Purchase one of the many fat-free dressings available (most still contain 25 to 50 calories) or use "spray on" salad dressing to lower your caloric intake.

Day 7 – Find a favorite snack food that's low in fat: light popcorn, bite-size pretzels, low-fat string cheese, fresh fruit or veggies, and frozen fruit-juice bars.

WEEK 13

Habits that Help

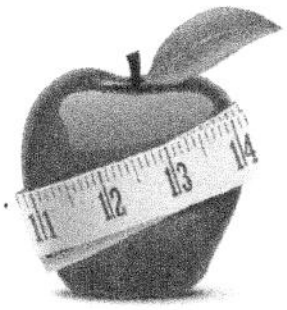

YOU'VE HEARD IT time and again: It takes 21 days to develop a habit. Why not try it and see? Take 21 days to develop just one good weight loss habit. It might be eating fresh fruit for dessert, deciding to eat a healthy breakfast each day, or waking up 15 minutes earlier for a brisk walk.

Let's face it—we all have good habits and bad habits. Many began in childhood. One that most people can relate to is eating dessert after a meal. If you don't have dessert, you don't feel satisfied and want something more. Wanting more leads to nighttime eating that can mean extra calories you don't need. Another habit is eating in front of the television. Some people can consume as much as an extra meal's worth of calories when they eat in front of the TV. It's termed "mindless eating" because you are not really aware of your intake. Be aware of every bite. Small bites add up quickly. See the example below:

Time of Day	Food/behavior	Calories
8:00 a.m	¼ cup of orange juice remains in the carton. You choose to drink it rather than put that small amount back in the refrigerator	28
8:05 a.m	You still have milk in your bowl, so why not add a little more cereal to use it up? (extra ¼ cup cereal)	50
10:00 a.m	You need a pick-me-up at work, but the coffee tastes too strong. You add 2 Tbsp. of fat-free coffee creamer	50
12:30 p.m	You ordered your lunch salad with dressing on the side, but it mistakenly came with dressing on it, and you decide to eat it anyway. (1 extra Tbsp. of dressing)	55
2:00 p.m	Pop two small pieces of chocolate into your mouth from the office candy bowl.	50
5:00 p.m	Eat a small handful of snack crackers while preparing dinner.	80
6:30 p.m	There's a bit of rice left from dinner. It's barely enough to save, so you opt to eat the last ½ cup.	108
9:00 p.m.	You pop a slice of cheese in your mouth while making lunches for tomorrow	113
	Total	534

All these little extras added up to 534 calories. As previously stated, an extra 500 calories each day can cause a one-pound-per-week weight gain. Often the little extras are what lead to weight gain in most people. The good news is that small changes can lead to weight loss as well.

Addiction experts have found that even hard-core addicts can successfully break their long-term, life-threatening, bad habits by just cutting back little by little instead of trying to quit all at once. That means setting up a regimen of moderation rather than total abstinence. Successful moderation means deciding in advance how much is "too much" and then making sure you stick to that limit no matter what. Take time to map out your eating habits. Identify the ones that you could improve using the guidelines in this book develop strategies to transform that bad habit into a good one.

Questions to Consider:

- Do I automatically want dessert after a meal?
- Can I watch TV without eating?

Day 1 – Brush your teeth right after dinner. It symbolizes that your mouth and the kitchen are closed for business.

Day 2 – Tape a note to the refrigerator that says, "Not tonight," or, "Am I really hungry?"

Day 3 – If you "snack," choose one that's healthy and takes time to eat, such as a salad with light dressing, a bag of light popcorn, or a bowl of high-fiber cereal (e.g. bran flakes or oatmeal) and fat-free milk.

Day 4 – Because snacking is often done to reduce stress, try relaxation techniques instead.

Day 5 – Find something else you like to do such as play solitaire, knit, or read and try this activity rather than watching TV and eating.

Day 6 – Don't deprive yourself all day long; otherwise, you'll for sure want to snack at night when your self-control isn't as strong after a hectic day.

Day 7 – Pick one bad habit to change and start counting off your 21 days today.

WEEK 14
Be Committed

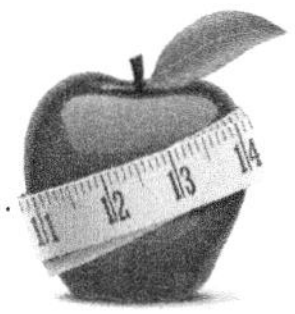

MAKING A FIRM commitment is probably one of the most important steps a person needs to take on his or her journey to weight loss. If you are not committed, it just won't happen, at least not for the long term. You can't roll out of bed one morning and decide to lose fifty pounds in two months. It just doesn't happen that way. You need to take time to think it through, make a realistic plan, and then work the plan.

The word "work" is key. Weight loss is not easy. Reaching almost any goal (getting a diploma from high school or college, getting a promotion at work, saving for a new car or a first home) is not easy. But look back over your life and you'll see that you've indeed reached many goals, most of which were not easily attained. With a committed attitude, you can reach your weight loss goal. Many psychologists say that writing your commitment down helps solidify it in your mind. A written statement makes your plans concrete and keeps you moving in the right direction.

In 2011 the American Dietetic Association surveyed 754 people nationwide and asked them why they did not eat a balanced diet. They gave the following responses:

- 82% – I don't want to give up the foods I like.
- 62% – It takes too much time to keep track of my diet.
- 47% – I need more practical tips to help me eat right.
- 40% – I don't know or understand guidelines for diet and nutrition.

Some of those responses may be familiar to you. This book provides you with the tools you need for weight loss. All you need to bring is the commitment.

Questions to Consider:

- How many times in the past have I wanted to lose weight but have not been committed to it?
- Am I ready to "work" at weight loss?

Day 1 – Make a list of other commitments and successes you have accomplished.

Day 2 – Review your list of past accomplishments and record how much time they took to complete. Realize that your path to genuine weight loss will also take time and commitment.

Day 3 – Make a list of all the reasons you want to lose weight. Are you losing weight for yourself or because someone else wants you to lose weight?

Day 4 – Write down your commitment to weight loss in definite terms. (See Week 18 on setting goals.) Post it someplace you'll see it every day.

Day 5 – Make a realistic plan to bring your commitment to a successful finish.

Day 6 – Look at what you have already accomplished using the weight loss advice found in one of the previous chapters. You committed to that objective, so you can commit to another one.

Day 7 – Look for friends or relatives who will help you stay committed.

WEEK 15

Get NEAT

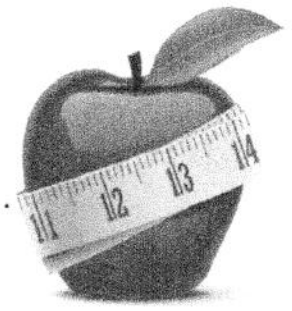

THE ACRONYM NEAT stands for non-exercise activity thermogenesis. This means that any movement we make takes energy or burns calories. Someone with way too much time on his or her hands figured out that if a person chews gum 24 hours a day for an entire year, that person will lose 10 pounds. Of course, no one could chew gum 24 hours a day for an entire year, but it does speak to the fact that any amount of movement burns calories. So, if you apply this concept to weight loss, all you have to do is **move more**.

NEAT activity can vary greatly. Even minor changes in physical activity throughout the day could increase your total calorie burn by 20 percent. The Mayo Clinic College of Medicine under the direction of Dr. James Levine has studied NEAT for both lean and mildly obese groups. Interestingly enough, they found that lean participants moved 2.5 more hours a day than the mildly obese. Moving included standing or just plain fidgeting. They found that standing instead of sitting could possibly burn 10 percent more calories.

Exercise is not a free pass to eat more. A 1.5 ounce chocolate bar = 35 minutes of biking.

During studies at the Mayo Clinic, participants were asked to wear custom-made, data-logging undergarments 24 hours a day that monitored every wiggle made during their normal daily regimen. They found that people who tapped their feet, preferred to stand rather than sit, and generally moved more burned up to 350 more calories per day. That alone could add up to a 37-pound weight loss in a year. The Mayo team suggests our modern society has eliminated many labor-intense activities that may be to blame for the increased weight most people carry. For instance, we don't shovel snow anymore, we snow blow it; we don't wash dishes standing by the sink anymore, the automatic dishwasher does it for us; we don't take the stairs anymore, we use elevators or escalators. Actually, the Mayo Clinic studies show that it might be more effective to achieve a healthy body weight by increasing NEAT in your life than to seek a form of organized exercise. So let's look at the WOW days below to see how we can incorporate more movement into each day.

Questions to Consider:

- Do I take the stairs whenever possible?
- Do I look for the parking place closest to the store so that I don't have to walk?
- Can I shovel snow or rake leaves rather than blow them?

WoW
Working on Weight Loss

Day 1 – When you talk on the phone today, stand up. (Don't sit down.)

Day 2 – Set the timer on your watch or phone and, every half hour, walk around the office or house.

Day 3 – While sitting at your desk or lunch table, wiggle/tap your feet under it.

Day 4 – When singing hymns at church before or during the service, step side to side in time to the music.

Day 5 – Stand on the subway or bus rather than sit. March in place while brushing your teeth.

Day 6 – Pace back and forth in front of the TV as you watch the half hour evening news.

Day 7 – Step side to side as you wait in line to buy tickets at the movies, the ball game, or the theater.

WEEK 16

Move More

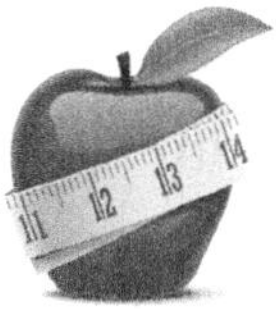

JUST AS YOU find time for brushing your teeth, make activity a part of every day. Often we skip exercise because we don't have a one-hour block of time to dedicate to the gym. We need to take care of ourselves and find time for exercise. As many trainers will tell you, the best exercise is the one you will regularly do. Try various activities such as walking, cycling, or swimming and see what you like best. Be sure to vary your routine. Most trainers recommend cross-training because it helps keep you from getting bored, and it causes you to use different muscles which can help prevent injury. If you enjoy walking, that is great. To cross-train, simply add some strength or resistance activities throughout the week, such as pushups and lunges. The higher the intensity of the workout (the harder you work) the more calories you burn.

Exercise helps you build muscle. As muscle mass increases, your metabolic rate should also increase, which means you will burn more calories. As you increase muscle, you may see some weight gain because muscle is denser than fat. However, if you are exercising and not seeing weight loss, don't automatically attribute it to an increase in muscle. It takes about one month to see a significant change in muscle mass. Reevaluate your weight loss plan, make changes if necessary, and have patience.

You win... if you don't quit.

If you are a beginner to exercise, start with 50 minutes of exercise a week (10 minutes a day for five days) and work up to your goal. A good goal for most people is a minimum of 30 minutes of moderate to vigorous activity most days. To reach a healthy weight, you may need to be physically active for a longer period of time—as much as 60 to 90 minutes a day—or participate in more intense activities. Any time you are beginning an exercise program, it is wise to consult a doctor for medical clearance.

Working out an extra 60 minutes weekly (just 10 minutes, six days a week) could help burn three times more fat, according to a study in the *Journal of Strength and Conditioning Research*. People who did a half hour of cardio twice weekly lost four pounds of fat over eight weeks, while those who did four sessions a week lost a whopping 13 pounds. It is also possible they were able to keep their goals at the forefront because they were exercising more frequently, so perhaps they ate better as well.

The calories burned during exercise are affected by body weight, intensity of workout, individual conditioning level, and metabolism. The values below are estimates of what it would take to burn 200 calories based upon a 205-pound adult. See Appendix A for more activities.

- Vacuum for 32 minutes
- Wii Bowling for 46 minutes
- Golf (pulling clubs) for 21 minutes
- Walking (brisk pace of 3.5 mph) for 28 minutes

Tips to stay on track:

- Find an exercise buddy whom you are compatible with—don't choose a friend who likes weight training in the evening if you prefer yoga in the morning.
- Find an activity you enjoy. Experiment with some of the following: go to the gym, use an exercise DVD, walk, bicycle, use a treadmill or elliptical machine, or go hiking.
- Schedule your exercise. Often, morning workouts are best simply because they are less likely to be interrupted. If you wait until afternoon or evening, things always seem to come up that take you away from your exercise time.
- Don't do too much, too fast. People who overdo it from the start frequently wind up with injuries and quit.
- After three weeks, look for improvements such as walking farther, less shortness of breath, or more flexibility. You will feel a sense of accomplishment to see your overall progress.

Remember, every little bit helps. Take your dog for a long walk; rake leaves rather than using the leaf blower; go for a bike ride with your children; take the stairs at home or work; park away from your destination when running errands. You may also want to try commercial calisthenics. Anytime you find yourself sitting and watching television, get up and walk around during the commercials or do calisthenics such as sit-ups, lunges, squats, or pushups. If you record your favorite shows and skip commercials, then do the calisthenics while watching your favorite show.

With the current childhood obesity epidemic, parents need to be active in order to be good role models for children. We frequently rush home from work, hurriedly put a "not so healthy" meal on the table, and then hop into the car to race to a sporting event (or to a meeting, or to the airport to catch a flight) where we ***sit*** for at least an hour. Instead of sitting that whole time, take a quick walk during your child's sporting event, in between meetings, or while waiting at the airport. Focus on being active. Any and all activity helps.

Questions to consider:

- Have I put myself and my exercise first today?
- What is my excuse for not exercising?
- Can I find an exercise that I truly enjoy?

Day 1 – Choose an activity and do it for 10 to 15 minutes this morning.

Day 2 – Try a new activity this week.

Day 3 – Take a walk during a work break even if it's just down the hall and back.

Day 4 – If you have mid-afternoon sleepiness, walk around to energize yourself rather than consuming a high-calorie food or drink.

Day 5 – Do commercial calisthenics tonight.

Day 6 – Take the stairs every chance you get today.

Day 7 – Exercise twice today for 15 minutes each time.

WEEK 17

Keep a Food Journal

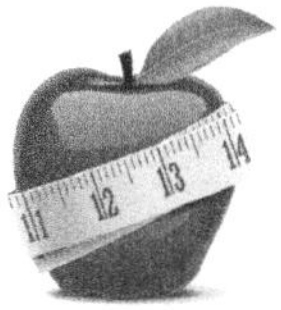

SURPRISINGLY, FOOD RECORDS are typically only 50 percent accurate. Why are they so unreliable? Most people don't record everything they eat or don't include actual or accurate portion sizes.

Then why keep a food journal? If you honestly keep track of your foods and your eating habits, the journal will help you identify areas that need work. It may be as simple as realizing you could significantly reduce caloric intake by using one tablespoon of low-fat salad dressing (25 to 35 calories) rather than four tablespoons of regular salad dressing (250 calories), or by substituting diet soda (zero calories for 12 ounces) for regular soda (150 calories for 12 ounces).

Are you recording food that you pop into your mouth while cooking, putting leftovers away, or packing lunches for yourself or the kids? If not, you need to. Also, keep track of why you are eating. Are you feeling deprived, tired, hungry, anxious, or are you unsure?

*Make short-term goals such as, two pounds per week, **not** 25 pounds by summer.*

Keep track of how a half cup of rice looks on your dinner plate or three-quarters of a cup of cereal in your home cereal bowl. You don't need to measure daily, but do a "visual measure" every time you eat.

Keep your food journal on paper, on a computerized worksheet, on a sound website, or perhaps on a smart phone application. There are multiple methods of keeping track of intake, but the bottom line is that you need to be honest in your record keeping or it won't help.

Questions to consider:

- Am I fooling myself with my journal or being honest?
- Can I see trends regarding when and where I eat the most?
- Am I eating because of physical hunger or emotional needs?

Day 1 – Measure everything you eat today. Pay attention to how it looks in a bowl or on a plate.

Day 2 – Record everything on paper, an online journal, or smart phone application.

Day 3 – Which of the foods that you recorded are the least healthy?

Day 4 – Which unhealthy foods would be easiest to limit or live without?

Day 5 – Change one poor food habit from the past four days.

Day 6 – Continue changing one bad habit from day five.

Day 7 – Did you make a significant difference in total calorie intake over the past two days? Was it a savings of more than 100 calories per day? Congratulate yourself!

WEEK 18
Be SMART

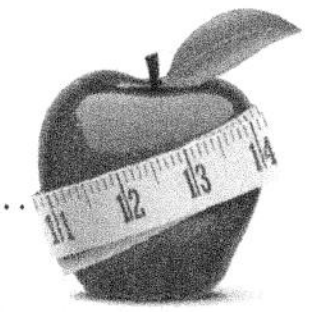

IF YOU DISCIPLINE yourself to get up each morning to go to work, or complete a project, or do the laundry each week, you can discipline yourself for weight loss. Having a plan will give you the discipline you need to develop new, healthy eating patterns. You need to have a plan with set goals so that it will carry you in the right direction even when you don't feel like following the plan. Your goals need to be focused, specific, and realistic. Writing down your goals will strengthen your potential for success because you can visualize the strategy. Writing them down will make them concrete rather than just vague dreams floating around in your head. Your realistic goals need to be measurable. A vague goal of "I will lose weight" can't be measured. Setting a goal to lose one to two pounds each week can motivate you to take steps to meet it.

Professional coaches often use the following questions to set effective goals.

SMART: (Specific, Measurable, Attainable, Realistic, Targeted)

- Are they **S**pecific? Identifying exactly what you want to accomplish helps you plan the steps that lead to your goal.
- Are they **M**easurable? Your goals should be concrete such as, five pounds in two weeks, so you can chart the progress you are making.
- Are they **A**ttainable? Set goals that are slightly out of your immediate grasp, but not so far that there is little or no hope of ever achieving them.
- Are they **R**ealistic? Losing 5 to 10 percent of your current weight may be a realistic goal for you.
- Are they **T**argeted? Having a clear objective, such as getting a new outfit one or two sizes smaller, should encourage your focus.

Questions to Consider:

- Do I set goals that are not realistic?
- Do I set my own goals that I think will work for me or try something I've read in the latest magazine article?
- Have I written down my goals?

Day 1 – Set exercise goals for three days this week and stick to them.

Day 2 – Plan to cut 100 calories from your daily meal plan for two days this week.

Day 3 – Determine to order thin crust pizza (two slices) instead of regular crust and save 140 calories.

Day 4 – Set a goal to walk up at least one flight of stairs each day rather than use the elevator.

Day 5 – Set a goal to give away or sell all your clothes that are now too big.

Day 6 – Determine to order wine or wine spritzers rather than calorie-laden mixed drinks.

Day 7 – Set a goal to get a pedometer and walk at least 2,000 steps each day.

WEEK 19

Weighing In

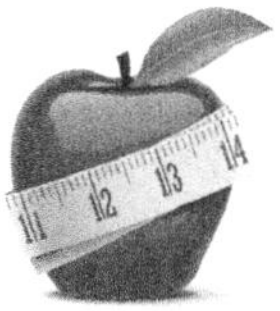

ONCE YOU RESOLVE to lose weight and are following a healthy plan, the question many people ask is, "To weigh or not to weigh?" The answer actually depends on the individual. Some people obsess over the numbers on the scale and weigh several times a day. This usually doesn't work well because your weight will fluctuate three to five pounds over the course of the day depending on how much you eat and drink and, for women, hormonal changes. Drink a 32-ounce glass of iced tea, and you just gained two pounds. For some people, weighing once a week is all they need. You can use other measures to identify if you have lost weight. You can tell if your jeans fit better without ever stepping on a scale. Perhaps you can use the next smaller hole on your belt.

A helpful number to measure is the size (circumference) of your waist. The unhealthiest place to carry extra weight is around your midsection. A high waist circumference and too much abdominal fat increase your risk of diabetes, high blood pressure, high cholesterol, and heart disease. If your waist circumference is greater than 40 inches in men or 35 inches in women, you may be at increased risk. To measure your circumference, place a tape measure around your bare abdomen just above your hip bone. Be sure that the tape is snug, does not compress your skin, and is parallel to the floor. Relax, exhale, and measure your waist.

Remember, digital and battery operated scales can give you skewed readings when batteries run low.

If you do decide to weigh daily, you should always use the same scale. It may not be exactly accurate, but it will give you the correct number of pounds you lose on any given day. In order to receive the most accurate information regarding your weight loss, weigh at the same time each day. You should weigh the least first thing in the morning after using the bathroom. You should also weigh yourself dressed in the same clothes each day, or, if you weigh first thing each morning, you may want to weigh in the nude. Once you reach your goal weight (and you will), weighing once a day is probably a good idea. One study showed that women who did weigh once each day were 82 percent less likely to regain the weight they lost.

Questions to Consider:

- Do I want to weigh after every meal?
- Do I weigh at the same time each day?

Day 1 – Put a new, five-pound bag of flour or sugar on your scale to check the calibration and adjust the scale accordingly.

Day 2 – Use the same scale you adjusted to weigh each time.

Day 3 – Check how your favorite pair of jeans fit today. Recheck that fit three weeks from now.

Day 4 – Take your favorite belt and note the proper fit now. Or measure your waist with a fabric tape measure. Once you've lost five pounds, check that fit or measure again.

Day 5 – Weigh at the same time each day to better assess your actual losses.

Day 6 – Determine to weigh no more than once a day.

Day 7 – Be sure you weigh in the same clothes each time you weigh.

WEEK 20

Fast Food Fixes

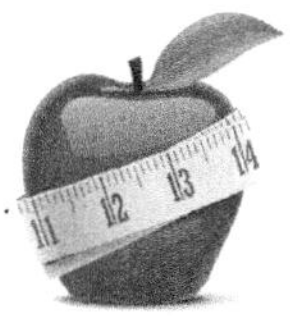

MANY DIETS WILL tell you to stay away from fast foods at all costs. Let's get real—with our busy schedules, it would be almost impossible to avoid fast food altogether. Instead, try looking at fast food in a new light. Number one, you really don't need to make it a routine stop several times a week. Number two, you don't need to order the double bacon cheeseburger with super-sized fries.

Today, most fast food establishments have healthier options available. Grilled chicken sandwiches, low-fat dressings, and fruit as a side rather than fries are just a few of the options available for a calorie-conscious person. If you really want to have a burger with fries, think kid-sized. A kid-sized burger with fries should come in at under 500 calories, and that will surely fit into your meal plan.

If you plan to select a fast food salad option, remember Caesar salads are packed with extra calories—choose a grilled chicken salad with low-fat dressing instead. Beware of anything "stuffed." That word means just what it says. The stuffed crust pizza is stuffed with extra cheese and calories as is the stuffed burrito. If you're looking for a quick summer treat, skip the chocolate milkshake and opt for a small, soft-serve chocolate cone instead; you'll save more than 100 calories.

At chicken restaurants, rather than ordering a chicken Caesar wrap (460 calories), choose chicken soup (140 calories), a char-grilled chicken salad (180 calories), and a small ice cream cone (150 calories) for a total of 470 calories. At a fast food Mexican restaurant, pass on the seven-layer burrito (490 calories) and instead choose a small taco (150 calories), a side of pinto beans with no cheese (110 calories), and one dessert cinnamon twist (170 calories) for a total of 430 calories. At the burger joint, instead of ordering a double cheeseburger (560 calories), choose a small hamburger (260 calories), a side salad (20 calories), and a small order of fries (250 calories) for a total of 530 calories. You'll receive the same number of calories, yet eat more food and feel more satisfied.

Questions to Consider:

- How often do I stop to eat at fast food establishments?
- Have I ever reviewed the menu choices to see if lower-calorie items are available?
- Do I choose coffee drinks loaded with whipped cream?

Day 1 – Take advantage of light mayo offered by some fast food places.

Day 2 – Order skinless chicken or take the skin off before eating. It saves both fat and calories.

Day 3 – Use BBQ sauce to add flavor to grilled chicken sandwiches to avoid the extra calories and fat found in mayonnaise and special sauces.

Day 4 – Ask for mustard or ketchup only, no mayonnaise or special sauces.

Day 5 – Pile on lettuce, tomato, onion, and dill pickles instead of cheese and bacon.

Day 6 – Swap out fries for dipping fruits or fruit cups.

Day 7 – Ask for whole wheat breads or tortillas to give you a healthier option.

WEEK 21

Designations for Dining Out

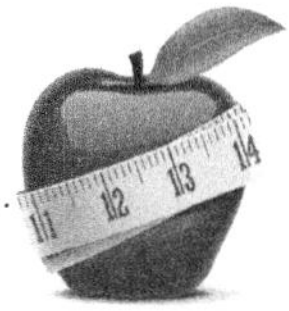

EATING OUT CAN be one of the biggest challenges for anyone trying to lose weight. For some, it's better to just cancel restaurant plans. However, that's no fun and who wants to never enjoy fine dining? By following a few simple suggestions, you can enjoy the atmosphere, friends, and the food.

If you're finished with your meal & don't plan to take any home, pour salt on the food so that you won't be tempted to eat more.

First, never go out to eat when you're starving. Eat something at home like a few whole wheat crackers or half an apple to take the edge off. While you are reviewing the menu, opt for water with lemon rather than an alcoholic beverage. Many mixed drinks can add 200 to 500 calories to your meal. Light beer has about 100 calories in a 12-ounce can or bottle and just five ounces of red or white wine has about 100 to 125 calories. Five ounces of sweet dessert wine will be close to 250 calories. Additionally, alcohol may lessen your ability to make wise choices.

Look at the menu carefully. If the words *crispy* or *crunchy* appear, that means the item is likely fried, so continue looking. Search for the words *baked*, *broiled*, *grilled*, *roasted*, *steamed*, or *poached*. These cooking methods will provide meats or veggies that contain far fewer calories. Make sure items are prepared without gravies or sauces. Order a plain baked potato, not loaded, and ask for butter and sour cream on the side so that you can portion wisely. Two tablespoons of sour cream is 51 calories while two tablespoons of butter or margarine equals about 200 calories. If a bread basket appears, look for the whole wheat roll and limit yourself to one. Try to avoid biscuits or croissants. (One dinner roll is about 75 calories, one biscuit comes to about 125 calories, and a croissant is closer to 225 calories.) When establishments serve chips and salsa prior to a meal and you know you can't resist, ask the waiter not to bring them to your table.

Questioning what a menu item is? You won't know if you don't ask. If the waiter tells you the item is pan-fried, ask to have it prepared another way. Don't be afraid to customize your order. Ask for cottage cheese or a salad instead of fries. Vegetarian selections could be lower in calories, so don't overlook them. Side items such as steamed vegetables and a cup of broth-based soup could also be combined into a healthy, balanced, low-calorie meal. The kids' menu does not necessarily mean smaller portions. Some may be large portions of foods that are high in fat and calories. An entrée salad may or may not be a wise choice.

Enormous salads with high-calorie additions such as sweetened dried fruit, nuts, croutons, chips, and salad dressing are not good. You might also consider ordering a smaller appetizer portion of an entrée or a side salad as a meal.

If a salad comes with your meal, you have several options. You can order it plain with lemon. Squeeze the lemon generously on the salad and lightly salt it. One other way to enjoy a salad with dressing is to order the dressing on the side. Then, rather than portion it out, dip your fork into the dressing then into the salad. You'll get full flavor, but only a smidgeon of the calories. A small side salad without dressing would average around 50 to 60 calories if it contained shredded cheese. A side salad with only vegetables and no cheese or croutons would average closer to 25 to 30 calories. A Caesar salad would be close to 300 calories because all those healthy greens are coated with a dressing made of oil and eggs plus croutons and Parmesan cheese.

Questions to Consider:

- Do I look for new and interesting menu items at my favorite restaurant?
- Do I always order an appetizer?
- Do I enjoy the food or the fellowship more at restaurants?

Day 1 – Determine to always ask for salad dressing on the side.

Day 2 – Divide an entrée with your partner to automatically cut your calories in half.

Day 3 – Try herbal tea or coffee for dessert.

Day 4 – If you can't resist dessert, order one that's mostly fruit and split it two or three ways.

Day 5 – Go for marinara sauce, not Alfredo.

Day 6 – Order steamed brown rice, not fried rice, with oriental entrees.

Day 7 – Beware of appetizers. Just one batter-dipped fried onion could total as much as 2,150 calories.

WEEK 22
Sleep Tight

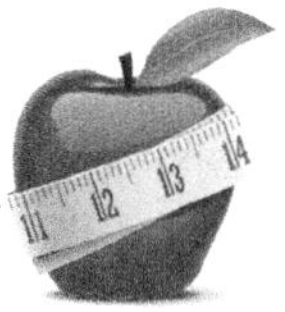

THE MORE UNINTERRUPTED sleep you get the better because the rapid eye movement and slow-wave sleep patterns are so restorative. Studies show that men need an optimal seven to eight hours of sleep each night, and women need six to seven hours—and these should be solid hours. Science tells us that it takes 2.5 hours of continuous sleep before it becomes truly restorative. Science also tells us that lack of sleep triggers hormonal shifts that may boost hunger and appetite. Researchers also speculate that lack of sleep may somehow slow down metabolism so that people burn fewer calories around the clock.

Bright light from a TV or computer screen can disturb your body's natural sleep-wake cycles and stimulate your nervous system. Adjusting the brightness setting of your TV or computer at least a half hour before

Avoid caffeine at least three hours before going to sleep. Some people may need to avoid it eight hours before bedtime.

retiring may help. The light from a digital clock may also make your room too bright, and, if you wake up, glance at the clock, and panic because of the time, you may have trouble falling back to sleep. Ignoring a lack of sleep is like ignoring a leaky faucet—if you do nothing, things will only get worse.

Questions to Consider:

- How many hours of sleep do I get on average?
- Is my sleep continuous?
- Do I put off bedtime to finish a task or project?

WoW Working on Weight Loss

Day 1 – Dim the lights 20 minutes before bedtime to help you relax.

Day 2 – If you have trouble falling asleep, try reading in bed until you feel drowsy. (Be picky about your reading material—no novels you "can't put down.")

Day 3 – Get into a relaxing bedtime routine and make a normal bedtime the rule rather than the exception.

Day 4 – Make a list of things you'll do tomorrow so that they will be off your mind and not keep you awake.

Day 5 – Noisy partner? Try ear plugs for yourself or non-snoring remedies for your partner.

Day 6 – Make sure your room is dark.

Day 7 – For two mornings in a row, wake up without an alarm. However long you sleep is probably how much you require.

WEEK 23

Get a Grasp on Groceries

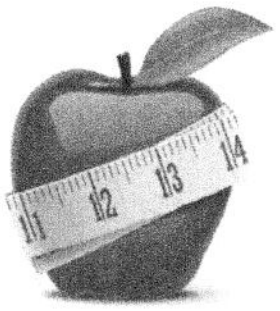

ANYTIME YOU ARE trying to become healthier, you need to look at your grocery shopping habits. You don't really need to go to a specialty store to get healthy foods. However, you do need to take a good hard look at your current habits. Probably the first and foremost tip is to never shop when you are hungry. If you do, everything will look good, and you'll likely buy unhealthy as well as healthy items. So munch on an apple, banana, or a slice of whole wheat bread spread with peanut butter before you make your routine run to the neighborhood grocery.

In addition, always use a list. It could be one you make throughout the week as you notice items you need. It could be one from a website that gives you menu ideas for the week, but by using a list, you'll be less tempted to purchase "impulse items."

Don't compare yourself to others. Focus on your own accomplishments.

As mentioned in Week 4, "Making Sense of Nutrition Labels", it is best to find the healthiest option for each food item on your list. Cereals are an example of a set of items that run the gamut from healthy to very unhealthy. Remember, you only need to read a few labels in that section once to determine which items would be best.

Questions to Consider:

- Do I make emergency runs to the grocery store and come home with more items than necessary?
- Do I shop with a list most of the time?
- Can I read nutrition labels?

Day 1 – Take time to read nutrition labels today in one section (e.g. spaghetti sauce). Then do a section once a week to learn which items are the healthiest.

Day 2 – Shop the perimeter of the store. Usually items placed along the outside walls are the healthiest. This would include fresh fruits and veggies, milk and other low fat dairy products, meats, and sometimes frozen foods and breads. The aisles are more often than not packed with chips, soda pop, cookies, crackers, and many other high-fat and high-sugar foods.

Day 3 – Don't give in to coupons. Just because you found a $1.00 coupon doesn't mean you need to purchase that item. Stop and think, is it healthy? Do I really need it? Will I really use it?

Day 4 – If today is grocery-shopping day—take a list and eat a snack before going. Never shop while hungry.

Day 5 – Try a store brand that's lower in cost. It may be just as high quality as a name brand. You only have to purchase the item once to determine if it will work for you. If you really don't like the store brand, go back to your name brand.

Day 6 – When you're checking out labels, if it has more than five items that you've never heard of and can't pronounce, think twice before buying it.

Day 7 – Check out menu-planning websites. Most have healthy options which can simplify your grocery shopping and menu planning. Some sites require a fee to subscribe, but others offer suggestions at no cost.

WEEK 24

Choose Complex Carbohydrates

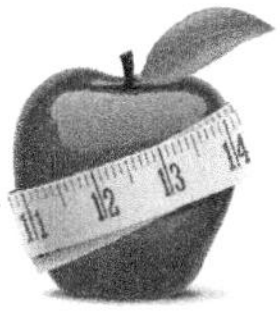

EATING THE RIGHT kind of carbohydrates (starches) may help you lose weight. Many studies suggest that eating high-fiber, low-calorie whole grains (complex carbohydrates) helps you avoid overeating and thus avoid weight gain. As mentioned before, no one diet fits everyone. However, most research studies agree that, in the long run, eating a varied diet that is low in calories and high in nutrients is the best way to lose weight with the added benefit of improving your heart and overall health.

Foods rich in complex carbohydrates tend to be low in fat and contain less sugar, so they can promote weight loss. In addition, they create a feeling of fullness and can delay hunger. It's best to get your fiber from foods, not fiber supplements. Foods with fiber provide nutrients such as vitamins, minerals, and antioxidants, and, therefore, give you much more than fiber. Selecting whole grain products, legumes (beans and peas), fruits, and vegetables instead of fiber supplements will benefit your overall health.

> *Watch a funny movie. People who watched a sad movie ate 30% more buttered popcorn than when they watched a happy film.*

Researchers usually divide fiber into two groups. Soluble fiber is found in legumes, nuts, oat bran, and many fruits and vegetables. It helps reduce your cholesterol levels and slows stomach emptying. Therefore, it helps protect your heart and can make you feel full longer, aiding in appetite control. The second group is called insoluble fiber and can be found in whole grain breads and cereals, flaxseeds, and the skins of many fruits and vegetables. Insoluble fiber helps keep you regular. The average person gets around 10 grams of fiber each day, but the recommended intake is 20 to 35 grams per day.

When you decide to increase your overall fiber intake, do it slowly. Increasing your intake too fast can cause gastrointestinal (GI) discomfort, including increased gas production or diarrhea. To prevent such problems, increase your fiber intake gradually over several weeks to give your GI tract time to adjust. Drinking plenty of fluids to soften the fibers as they move down the GI tract is also necessary. Finally, you can get your fiber from a variety of sources including fruits, vegetables, legumes, and whole grain breads, cereals, and pastas.

Questions to Consider:

- Do I regularly eat fiber-rich foods now?
- If not, why don't I eat more fiber? Am I afraid of GI discomfort?

Day 1 – If you don't like high-fiber cereal, gradually switch by mixing half high-fiber cereal (bran flakes) with half your usual cereal (frosted flakes).

Day 2 – To add fiber to muffins or pancakes, sprinkle a tablespoon of flaxseed into the batter. It adds a nutty flavor and one tablespoon of ground flaxseed provides a little more than three grams of fiber and only 55 calories.

Day 3 – Check the label on your wheat bread. Many manufacturers add caramel coloring to give their bread the appearance of being healthier. Look for 100 percent whole wheat flour as the first ingredient.

Day 4 – Add a can of beans or legumes to your soups or chili. Chickpeas make a great addition to tortilla soups and lentils will boost the fiber content of minestrone soup. Just half a cup of beans provides five to eight grams of fiber and about 100 calories.

Day 5 – Some companies are now making whole grain pasta that looks and tastes like the regular kind. Try it; you'll like it.

Day 6 – Iceberg lettuce is actually quite low in fiber. To boost your salad's fiber add sliced strawberries, sliced pears, or apples. Fresh fruit adds flavor, color, and boosts vitamins and minerals as well.

Day 7 – Try raw carrots with hummus for a snack instead of chips and dip. Just one cup of raw carrots provides three to four grams of fiber and only 50 calories.

WEEK 25

Positive is Powerful

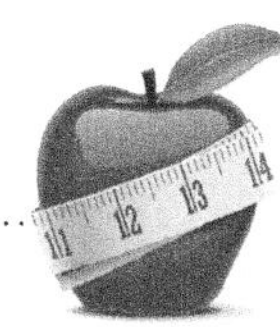

STUDY AFTER STUDY has found that an optimistic attitude, positive thinking, or affirmations can help people in many different areas. An old song once said, "Accentuate the positive and eliminate the negative." People would be much happier in life if they did that daily. When facing weight loss, that lesson is also true. Don't focus on how much weight you want to lose. Instead, focus on developing more healthy eating habits and becoming more active.

Having a positive perspective toward your health is better than a negative, self-sacrificing mindset when attempting to lose weight. Saying negative things about yourself will not make the weight come off any faster, but it might make you give up before you reach your goal. If you are constantly telling everyone that diets never work for you, you will actually begin to believe it. People cannot rise above their confessions so watch your confessions.

Rent a funny movie; laughter lowers stress & burns calories. One hour of laughter equals about a half hour of lifting weights.

The idea of making positive statements, affirmations, or declarations has been around since the early 1900s and has been the subject of many books, articles, and research. Positive thinking appears to protect your health by enhancing your immune system and encouraging an outgoing attitude, which can fend off anxiety and depression. Strong positive thinking and positive statements address two things: intention and anticipation. Intention is not just a desire or a hope; it brings about a determination to act. It focuses our attention, and, as we repeat our positive statements, we increase the likelihood of making those intentions a reality. Anticipation works in somewhat the same way. If you expect a good result, you actually filter incoming information in such a way that you are likely to get what you expect. Scientists call this the placebo effect. Researchers know that if a person expects a medication to work, it often will, even when it's just a sugar pill and not the real medicine.

To make positive thinking a part of your lifestyle, start small. Begin by saying, "I'm enjoying eating healthy foods," rather than, "I'm going to lose fifty pounds if it kills me." Find a statement you can truthfully say. Your statement needs to be a "want" not a "should." What matters is that you really, really want it. You also have to believe in the possibility of getting it. Your declarations should be expressed in the positive and present tense. Try, "I am losing weight," not, "I'll try again to lose weight." Lastly, voicing your positive statement out loud implies that you're committed to making it happen. Giving voice to your declaration is very powerful, and repetition helps. Just how many times a day you need to declare your positive phrase is up to you as there is no magic number, but hearing yourself repeat it will actually make you believe it.

Questions to Consider:

- Do I continually beat myself up with negative talk when I overeat?
- Are my weight loss declarations timid and wishful? "I *hope* I can do this."
- When I get dressed in the morning, do I let myself feel good about small changes in the way my clothes fit?

Day 1 – Begin each day with a positive statement. Say it out loud because it doubles the effectiveness.

Day 2 – Choose one battle to fight with a positive attitude. (Ignore the candy on your coworker's desk today.) When you choose your battles, you'll win them, and, eventually, you'll win the war on weight loss.

Day 3 – Don't focus on past failures; focus on new beginnings.

Day 4 – Make a list of positive statements that you can believe in and begin affirming them daily.

Day 5 – Post these positive statements around your home or office or car and read them out loud when possible.

Day 6 – Remember, no one is perfect. If you make a mistake, forgive yourself and start again.

Day 7 – If you believe, you'll receive; if you doubt, you'll do without.

WEEK 26

Negate Negative Thinking

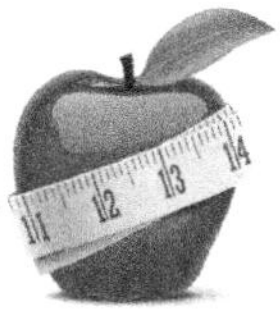

IT'S SAID THAT it takes 21 positives to overcome one negative. Now that's a lot of positives! Just think of all the negative statements you hear each day. The following story called "The Law of the Garbage Truck" illustrates how negative thinking and other negative issues affect us all.

One day I hopped in a taxi, and we took off for the airport. We were driving in the right lane when suddenly a black car swerved out of a parking space right in front of us. My taxi driver slammed on his brakes, skidded, and missed the other car by just inches. The driver of the other car whipped his head around and started yelling at us. My taxi driver just smiled and waved at the guy, and I mean, he was really friendly. So I asked, "Why did you just do that? That guy almost ruined your car and sent us to the hospital." This is when my taxi driver taught me what I now call, "The Law of the Garbage

Truck." He explained that many people are like garbage trucks. They run around full of garbage, full of frustration, full of anger, and full of disappointment. As their garbage piles up, they need a place to dump it, and sometimes they'll dump it on you. Don't take it personally. Just smile, wave, wish them well, and move on. Don't take their garbage and spread it to other people at work, at home, or on the streets. Life is 10 percent what you make it and 90 percent how you take it.

No doubt, a negative mentality can be the root of a negative reality. Negative thoughts are harmful to you. Neuroscientists know that our thought patterns create neural pathways in our brain. The more you "walk" down that negative path, the easier it is to go that way. The good thing is you can retrain your brain to think in a more positive way. Take notice of the messages your brain sends you each day. If you often find that the message is negative, switch channels when gloom and doom show up. Change to an optimistic and believable message.

Negative thoughts zap your energy big time. One way to feel energized is to list three things you're grateful for each day. A group of researchers asked people to do one of three things:

1. Keep a diary of what happened that day.
2. Record unpleasant experiences.
3. List the things for which they were grateful.

They found the grateful group had 25 percent more energy, slept better, and felt more enthusiastic. Switching from negative to positive thinking creates new pathways in your brain and becomes the new "way to go."

Questions to consider:

- Would people call me an optimist or a pessimist?
- Do I replay negative events in my mind?
- Do I look for the silver lining when things go wrong?

Day 1 – List three things for which you are grateful each day this week.

Day 2 – Go on a negative scavenger hunt; when you find something that brings you down, eliminate it. Perhaps it's the broken shade in the bedroom window or the weed that you haven't pulled up from the front walk or the pile of newspapers that never goes away in the front hall.

Day 3 – Think of one small thing you've wanted to do for some time and "do it."

Day 4 – Cuddle up with your partner, child, or pet (this should wash away those negative vibes).

Day 5 – Look for ways to make routine tasks fun. Put on some music and "move" with it as you vacuum. Sing some silly songs with the kids as you clear the dinner table or wash the car.

Day 6 – Try to "catch" other family members or friends making negative statements and make a game out of only "thinking positive."

Day 7 – Encourage positive conversations with friends and at work.

WEEK 27

Mind Your Munchies

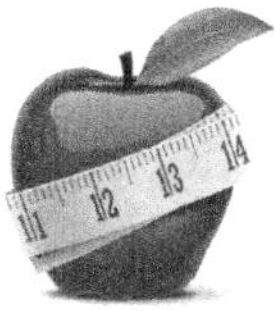

SNACKING CAN EITHER sabotage your new, healthy eating plan or give it new meaning. Eating every three to four hours (snacking) can ward off hunger and keep your metabolism revved up and your energy on an even keel. But don't confuse snacking with nibbling on high-fat and high-calorie goodies such as chips, cookies, and candy. To make snacking work for you, it needs to be planned into your weight loss strategy.

Plan to eat about five to six times a day with your snacks adding up to no more than 100 to 200 calories each. It's best to include some protein and fiber in your snacks as they will keep you feeling full longer. Feeling satisfied means you won't be as tempted to cheat. Actually, by planning two to three small snacks into your day, you'll be able to eat when you feel like it. You won't feel guilty because the snacks are planned. Snacking should give you more energy throughout the day and help prevent overeating.

Having cleaned out your pantry of unhealthy snacks like mini cheese crackers (30 = 150 calories) or chocolate sandwich cookies (2 = 130 calories), you need to replace them with healthier options. For example, one-quarter cup of peanuts is 200 calories and is a healthy option for a snack; one-quarter cup of soy nuts comes in at 100 calories and contains twice the calcium, almost twice the fiber, and slightly more iron. Mix the soy nuts with one-quarter cup dried cranberries, and you have a great snack for about 200 calories. Measure this mixture into plastic storage bags for an easy-to-carry snack for your office or auto. Refer to Appendix F for a list of more snacks that are about 50 to 100 calories each.

When you are feeling tempted to grab a high-calorie snack, focus on your goals in order to resist the urge. It only takes minutes to negate significant time spent exercising and eating healthy.

Questions to Consider

- What type of snacks am I now consuming?
- Do I eat meals at regular times?
- Do I use leftovers as snacks and consider their calories?

Day 1 – Check out the snacks you are eating. Decide if they are healthy. If not, find substitutes you can enjoy. Portion the unhealthy ones and enjoy them on special occasions.

Day 2 – Look at Appendix F and decide what snacks you would enjoy.

Day 3 – Hide unhealthy treats when you are storing food so that they are not in plain sight to tempt you.

Day 4 – Avoid vending machine snacks today.

Day 5 – Use "a million" layers of plastic wrap to store leftovers so that you'll be less tempted to cheat.

Day 6 – If you receive food items as gifts that are not on your snack plan, share them with friends so that you don't over indulge.

Day 7 – Don't go too long without eating. If you do, you'll be so hungry that you'll overindulge.

WEEK 28

Emotional Eating

FOOD IS OFTEN more than simple nourishment for our bodies. In most cultures, we offer food to show hospitality. Celebrations are often linked to food. Weddings, birthdays, and other celebrations typically involve food. While you were growing up, food may have been used as a reward, a punishment, or a diversion.

At times, all of us have eaten for emotional reasons. You may have been bored, happy, anxious, or sad. It is not a problem unless eating is the only coping strategy you have and if the foods you eat are unhealthy. However, if you frequently eat for emotional reasons and don't wait until you are hungry, you are very likely eating more than your body needs.

Some people are social eaters and lose sight of how much they consume while socializing. Review the chapter for Week 31, "Prepare for Parties", if this is your weakness. Still others eat to avoid disappointing a host. If you feel pressured to eat foods offered by friends or family, politely decline or try only a sample. The first bite will likely taste exactly the same as the twentieth bite—there is no need to overindulge.

Put down your fork between each bite. Women consumed almost 70 fewer calories when they took time to eat compared to eating quickly.

In Week 3 you learned about using a hunger scale. If you are an emotional eater, learning how to apply the hunger scale is important to your weight loss goals. If you find you are not hungry, you need a coping mechanism other than food to deal with the emotions you are feeling. See Appendix E for a list of things to do other than eat when you find yourself in such a situation. Additional ideas to assist in coping with emotional eating:

- Get plenty of sleep. It is easy to overeat in the hopes of gaining an energy boost.
- Avoid temptation. Keep trigger foods out of your home or work space.
- Don't starve yourself. Include healthy snacks throughout the day to avoid overeating at meals. Also, be sure to include some favorites so as not to feel deprived.
- Keep a food record of when/why/what you are eating.

Questions to Consider:

- Am I eating to feed my growling stomach or to feed a feeling?
- What foods always seem to comfort me?

Day 1 – Document when, why, and how much you eat today.

Day 2 – It's OK to allow yourself one treat today, just don't go overboard.

Day 3 – Remember, adequate sleep gives you energy for the day so that you don't depend on food to give you that extra burst each afternoon.

Day 4 – If you're stressed, try measures other than food to calm down.

Day 5 – Keep some healthy comfort foods handy so that you don't give in to unhealthy ones.

Day 6 – Take a 10-minute walk today and focus on all the positive aspects of your weight loss.

Day 7 – Look in the mirror this morning and tell yourself, "I can meet my weight loss goal."

WEEK 29

Permanent Changes, Over Temporary Fixes

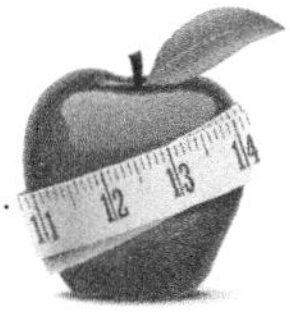

TEMPORARY FIXES SUCH as drinking a weight loss shake for breakfast and lunch each day are easy to follow for several weeks, perhaps even months. However, because they don't fit your lifestyle, it's easy to drop them and go back to a more comfortable way of doing things. To make weight loss work for the "long haul," you need to make permanent changes to your everyday life. These changes can range from eating breakfast every day to purchasing non-stick pans so that you can avoid tablespoons of high-calorie butter, margarine, or oils.

This book is all about taking ideas that make sense to you, applying them to your everyday life, and watching your weight drop gradually to a healthier you. To see your weight really come off and stay off, the changes you make need to be permanent. Therefore, the ideas you incorporate have to work for you, and you need to put some serious thought into which ones fit best. Review the following suggestions listed in other WOW sections:

- Use 100 percent whole wheat bread instead of white.
- If you can't give up energy drinks, choose one with fewer than 50 calories or limit yourself to one each day.
- Never skip meals as doing so slows down your metabolism.
- Drink plenty of fluids, as even mild dehydration can make you feel hungry.

Questions to Consider:

- Have I tried other "diets" that didn't fit my lifestyle?
- Am I committed to permanent changes and weight control, or am I just looking to lose weight for a special event?

WoW Working on Weight Loss

Day 1 – Buy nonstick cookware, use cooking spray or an oil mister in order to limit the amount of fat added while cooking.

Day 2 – Determine to always walk into the bank, dry cleaners, or pharmacy and not use the drive-through.

Day 3 – Decide to brush your teeth or gargle with mouthwash when a craving for ice cream or another favorite food hits. With a fresh mouth, you won't be so tempted to indulge.

Day 4 – Commit to permanently avoiding all vending machines that display your trigger foods.

Day 5 – Choose to allow only the 100-calorie pack, snack-type items into your pantry.

Day 6 – Resolve to surround yourself with people supportive of your commitment to weight loss rather than those who enable or encourage you to "cheat."

Day 7 – Elect to make activity a more permanent part of your lifestyle by making it a social event with family and friends just as you would with eating.

WEEK 30

Give Yourself a Break

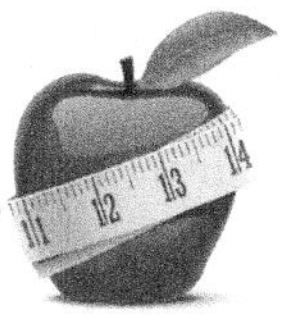

IT SEEMS AS if we usually encourage others but forget about ourselves. We give our time and energy to encourage our children in their school work or sporting activities, we encourage our partners, we give advice and encourage our co-workers or neighbors. But too often we give up when it comes to ourselves. It seems that we put everyone before us, even the dog or cat. However, in all honesty, we won't be there for our family and friends unless we take time to encourage ourselves and improve our overall health.

Your body is a valuable asset. Like a fine automobile it should be kept well-tuned. Treat yourself with respect and focus on the positive steps you have already taken. Try reminding yourself of how well you handled a situation last month when you turned down a great pastry at a restaurant, and you'll be better able to turn down an ordinary doughnut at the office. Another strategy to boost your spirits and willpower is to make a list of 10 things you're proud of, including items such as, "I get out of bed each day even when I don't want to do it," or, "I work well with everyone in the office." This will remind you of your strengths and what you can accomplish.

If your child does one thing wrong, you don't give up on them. You forgive them and help them get back on track. You should do the same for yourself. You *can* change your life for the better. You *can* reach your goals.

Questions to Consider

- When was the last time I spoke an encouraging word to myself?
- Do my actions show that I do consider myself valuable?
- Do I always put others ahead of myself?

Day 1 – Each morning, look in the mirror and repeat an encouraging statement such as, "I am losing weight," or, "I can walk twice as far as I did two weeks ago."

Day 2 – Take time to share with family and friends one thing you accomplished today.

Day 3 – Think of someone you encouraged today and how it improved their day. Now, think of something you can encourage yourself about today.

Day 4 – Take five minutes before you go (to work, to bed, to make dinner) to write down two encouraging statements about your weight loss.

Day 5 – Tell someone about an encouraging word you received today from a friend or family member.

Day 6 – Go for a walk to boost your energy and improve your mood.

Day 7 – Ask your family or friends to tell you an encouraging story about themselves.

WEEK 31

Prepare for Parties

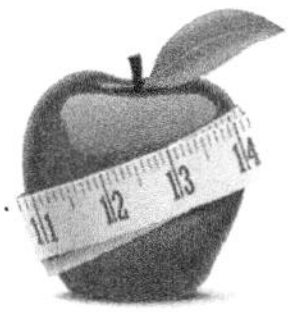

NAVIGATING YOUR WAY through office parties, family gatherings, and the various holiday seasons can be stressful, particularly when you are watching your weight. With proper planning, you can come through without added pounds showing up on your bathroom scale.

Proper planning means first, never leave for a party hungry. Always eat something about 30 to 60 minutes before leaving, or you'll be famished and ready to eat everything in sight. An apple or some whole wheat crackers with a piece of cheese are great pre-party snacks. On the way to the party do what professional athletes do—visualize how things will play out. See yourself skipping the high-calorie, high-fat *hors d'oeuvres* that you see at every party (e.g. pigs in a blanket) and select a healthier option (boiled shrimp with cocktail sauce). See yourself leaving the party satisfied and pleased with your control of the situation.

Because many parties are set up buffet style, let's look at that scenario. First, have a sparkling water with lemon or lime or with a splash of fruit juice to help fill you up with no calories. A six-ounce glass of wine will add 150 calories to the evening. Check out the buffet offerings before filling your plate. Grade the foods you really want to have (tasty or dessert-type items) from a 1 to 10 (10 being the best). Decide to select those foods that you grade as a 9 or 10 in reasonable portions. Pick the smallest plate available and fill two-thirds of it with vegetables and lean protein, leaving one-third for the "foods rated a 9 or 10." Holding out for the "10" foods gives you an edge. You will not feel deprived of that tasty treat, plus you can pat yourself on the back for not going over your calorie allotment.

Once your plate is full, move away from the buffet table. You won't be tempted to continue to nibble from the buffet and over-indulge. Another trick many people use is to have a prop at the party. If you are balancing a purse or a beverage, it becomes more difficult to eat. Savor every bite and enjoy conversations with others. It will give your brain a chance to tell you, "Hey, I'm satisfied now." You could try excusing yourself to the restroom about halfway through the party, again giving your brain a chance to tell you that you're full. If desserts are just too tempting and one little bite leads to another and another and another, you

Make pizza with veggie toppings. Try using broccoli, spinach, green or red peppers, tomatoes, mushrooms, or zucchini.

may want to skip desserts altogether. Instead, have a special treat such as low-fat frozen yogurt with fruit waiting for you when you get home. You can drizzle one tablespoon of chocolate syrup on top to really indulge for only 50 calories.

Questions to Consider:

- Do I automatically assume that I will gain weight over the holidays?
- Do I "save up" and not eat prior to the party so that I can indulge later?

Day 1 – When you have a party, give away all your "goodies" to other guests to take home.

Day 2 – Make a commitment to maintain your weight through the holiday season or when you are on vacation.

Day 3 – Focus on socializing rather than eating.

Day 4 – Remember, you can compromise and have one or two bacon wrapped scallops, then move to the boiled shrimp.

Day 5 – Remember, variety is the spice of life, but at a buffet you don't have to taste *everything* available.

Day 6 – If you love cheese, watch your portions. One ounce of sharp cheddar cheese is equal to 112 calories and one ounce of cream cheese has 101 calories.

Day 7 – Remember your middle school fractions and leave one-quarter of your plate for meat, like boiled shrimp or meatballs; one-quarter for a starch, like crackers or a wheat roll; and one-half of your plate for fruits and veggies.

WEEK 32

Strive for Five

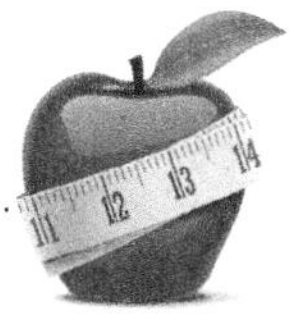

BY NOW, MOST of us understand the importance of eating more fruits and vegetables. They are low in calories and packed with vitamins, minerals, antioxidants, and phytochemicals. When compared with many people who consume only small amounts of fruits and vegetables, those who eat more generous amounts are likely to be a healthier weight and have a reduced risk of heart disease, high blood pressure, and diabetes.

Our lack of fruit and vegetable consumption often lies in the implementation phase. We sometimes don't want to purchase them because of the cost or fear of them going "bad" before we use them. If this is your fear, then buy small amounts of fresh produce or buy them frozen or canned. Frozen produce is typically flash-frozen at the peak of its freshness, and, if steamed,

Make a veggie wrap using roasted veggies and low fat cheese rolled in a whole wheat tortilla.

will retain valuable nutrients. When buying canned fruits, look for products packed in light syrup or fruit juice, not fruits packed in heavy syrup or with added sugars. Fruit packed in heavy syrup should be considered a dessert. Compare the following: one-half cup of fruit packed in natural juices has 62 calories while one-half cup canned fruit packed in syrup has 98 calories. Choose a variety of fruits and vegetables each day.

Now that you have purchased your fruits and vegetables, you need to eat them. Have them washed and ready to eat so that they take no more time to prepare than a convenience snack item. According to the Dietary Guidelines for Americans, adults should eat five servings of fruit and vegetables daily. A typical serving of fruits and vegetables is one-half cup.

Overall, available data suggests that eating more fruits and vegetables may be a useful part of programs designed for weight loss. Fruits and vegetables are high in water and fiber content and, therefore, low in calories. Fruits and vegetables may promote a feeling of fullness and decrease calorie intake. Therefore, it is reasonable to believe that diets rich in fruits and vegetables might prevent weight gain and lead to weight loss.

Questions to Consider:

- Do I currently eat five servings of fruits and vegetables daily?
- What prevents me from consuming enough fruits and vegetables?
- How can I make changes to incorporate more fruits and vegetables into my daily eating plan?

WoW
Working on Weight Loss

Day 1 – Add fresh or frozen fruit to your cold cereal, yogurt, pancake, or waffle. Add raisins to oatmeal.

Day 2 – Slice a vegetable (cucumbers or green peppers) to put on your sandwich today.

Day 3 – Have a cup of vegetable soup for a light lunch or as an afternoon snack.

Day4 – Add a grated vegetable to a sauce or casserole.

Day 5 – Try edamame as an appetizer, snack, or added to a salad. The soybean is flavorful, low in fat, and high in protein and provides fiber and vitamins. However, soybeans are not calorie-free: one cup of soybeans in the pods (one-half cup edible portion) provides 110 calories, nine grams protein, and three grams of fiber.

Day 6 – Eat a vegetable at breakfast. Try a grilled tomato or put red and green peppers in an omelet.

Day 7 – Add color and flavor to sandwiches with sliced pineapple, apple, or tomato as fillings.

WEEK 33

Use Self-Control

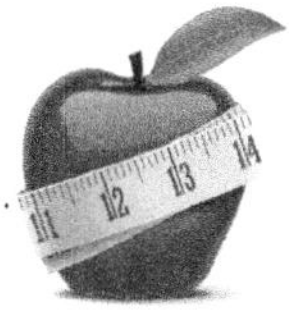

MOST PEOPLE CAN remember days when they were so busy that they didn't have time to eat a meal. When things slowed down, they were famished. Your body may have been telling you to eat, but your mind was too overwhelmed with other activities. Therefore, pay attention to what you are thinking. If you are constantly thinking about food, you are probably overeating, or you could be cutting your calories so drastically that your body is screaming for some nourishment. Neither scenario is good.

First you need to check your hunger scale (Week 3) to see if you truly need to eat. If you are hungry, eat. Having healthy snacks or meals on hand (at work, at home, or in the car) makes selecting the right food easier. Next, check your thinking (Weeks 25 and 26). What you program into your mind, you will ultimately believe; what you ultimately believe is what you will ultimately receive. If you believe you don't have time to watch your weight, you won't;

if you think you'll never be at a healthy weight, you won't. As the saying goes, "If you think you can't, you're right."

We also know that information overload can infringe on our decision-making powers. The same is true for our eating. Too much information in the form of a number of snacks in the pantry, breads or other goodies sitting on the kitchen counter, or platters overflowing with food on the dinner table all make it difficult for our brain to make rational, self-controlled choices. Your kitchen can actually set the mood for increased food consumption. But you can change the contents of your counters, pantry, or refrigerator to assist you in making healthy choices. Check out the suggestions in this WOW section.

Questions to Consider:

- Do I eat the right foods, but eat more than I planned?
- Do I rarely have time to cook and therefore grab anything convenient?
- Do I always eat when I'm frustrated, lonely, or bored?

WoW Working on Weight Loss

Day 1 – Take any unhealthy snack items off the kitchen counter, replacing them with healthy fresh fruits, and store ready-to-eat veggies in the refrigerator.

Day 2 – Keep only one kind of "treat" on hand at any given time. Limit yourself to a certain amount per day.

Day 3 – When in doubt, choose whole fruit over juice. It's more satisfying because it takes longer to eat, and it saves calories. Eating one-half of a grapefruit rather than drinking one eight-ounce glass of orange juice saves nearly 60 calories.

Day 4 – Stop and think before eating. Are you eating because you are tired or anxious, or are you truly hungry?

Day 5 – Forget large serving bowls. It's too tempting to go for seconds or thirds.

Day 6 – Package leftovers after plating the meal. Put them in single-serving containers for later.

Day 7 – Use smaller plates. A 10- to 12-inch plate needs lots of food to fill it up. When you use a smaller luncheon plate, your mind will see the full plate, and you'll be more satisfied. In the 1950s, the average plate size was 9 inches. In the 1980s, the average plate size was 11 inches. Today, the average plate size is 13 inches.

WEEK 34

Purge Your Pantry

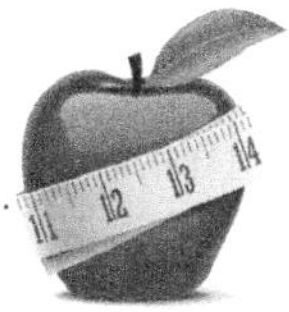

DON'T TEMPT YOURSELF with foods you shouldn't eat. It is much easier to resist an unhealthy, tempting food during a weak moment when it would require driving somewhere to get it rather than simply going to a shelf in your pantry. If you choose to keep some treats on hand for you or your family, be sure you limit them. Buy single-serving portions to reduce the likelihood of overindulging. If you buy in bulk, package items such as chips, crackers, nuts, and dried fruits into single servings before you store them.

Always have plenty of healthy foods, such as fruits and vegetables, readily available. When you buy fruits, wash a few as soon as you get home from the grocer. If fruits and vegetables are washed and ready to eat they will be just as "quick" as another option. For example, if you are in a hurry and need a quick snack, which is the better choice?

2 ounces of chips = 300 calories

OR

1 fresh apple, medium = 75 calories

Choosing chips rather than the apple will cost you an additional 225 calories. If you want to burn the additional calories, it will require almost an extra hour of walking time. So, then you have to ask yourself, *Did I really save myself any time by choosing the "quick" option?*

Questions to Consider

- What could I do today to reduce my calorie intake?
- Why do I have unhealthy foods in my home?
- Can I get into the habit of trading junk food for a fruit or vegetable?

Day 1 – Look in your pantry—pre-portion any chips, cookies, crackers, or unhealthy trigger foods.

Day 2 – Take a second look in your pantry. Is there a healthier option available, such as unsweetened canned fruit, low sugar cereal, baked chips, olive oil or canola oil? Add these healthier options to your grocery list.

Day 3 – Look in your refrigerator—are there healthier options available such as skim milk, fat-free sour cream, light salad dressings? Once again, add them to your grocery list.

Day 4 – Look in your freezer. Check out convenience items. Are they low-calorie, low-fat or low-sodium? Are the meats lean? Do you have any frozen treats such as ice cream? If so, is there a healthier option such as low-fat ice cream or frozen yogurt? Italian ice or fruit ice is typically a healthier choice than regular ice cream.

Day 5 – How many fruits do you have in your home (fresh, frozen, canned)—keep at least three on hand.

Day 6 – How many vegetables do you have in your home (fresh, frozen, canned)—keep at least three on hand.

Day 7 – Do you have plenty of whole grain foods? Healthy examples include whole wheat bread, whole grain pasta, rice, and legumes.

WEEK 35

Any Time Change is Desired, Work is Required

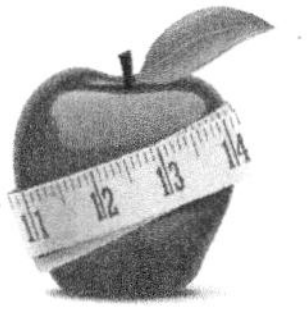

DESPITE SOME OF the weight loss claims in the media, long-lasting and healthful weight loss requires planning, patience, and persistence. It did not take one week to gain ten extra pounds, and, likewise, those ten pounds will not come off in one week. Nonetheless, people are drawn to the quick fixes reported for fad diets and weight loss pills. They are marketed to the public promising fabulous results with very little effort. However, quick fixes are unrealistic and usually short-lived. Slow, steady weight loss can be sustained, unlike dramatic weight changes. Healthy weight loss plans aim for a loss of one or two pounds per week. If you lose too quickly, you are likely losing muscle and water rather than fat. You are also more likely to regain the pounds.

There are no magic bullets—there are no foods or pills that magically melt or burn fat. No foods or pills will change your genetic makeup. There is no sound research showing that specific combinations of foods will aid in weight loss. You will need to move more and eat less to attain and maintain a healthy weight. Think about previous weight loss efforts you've tried. Why weren't they successful, or, if they were successful, how long did the results last? Think about what measures create long-lasting results.

Strive for progress, not perfection

Successful, long-term weight loss requires planning. You need a plan to fit your personal lifestyle. If there are not enough hours in the day for meal planning and exercise, how can you make it fit? You will need to prioritize. Perhaps there are some household duties you can delegate or postpone. If you come home famished most evenings without a plan for dinner, it may be difficult to consistently choose the healthiest options. You will most likely pick the quickest, easiest option that may or may not be healthy.

Take time to plan meals with a grocery list. Include lunch items on your list in order to avoid eating out for lunch most days. Purchase groceries in advance so that you are not scrambling at the last minute or shopping when you are hungry. Plan healthy meals that are easy to prepare and use basic ingredients that you already keep on hand. There are cookbooks and websites to assist you in preparing healthy meals in under thirty minutes. See Week 10, Enjoy Breakfast Every Day, for ideas on how to start your day.

Here are some simple changes to make:

- Steer clear of high-calorie beverages such as soda pop, energy drinks, specialty coffees, and alcohol.
- Eat slowly. It takes at least 20 minutes for your brain to signal that you are full, so slow down to avoid overeating.
- Plan time for meal preparation.
- Plan time for exercise.

Questions to Consider:

- Am I willing to work at losing weight, or am I hoping for quick, easy results?
- How many times have I tried to lose weight in the past? Why did I fail?
- How can I incorporate healthy eating and exercise into my lifestyle? What needs to change?

WoW Working on Weight Loss

Day 1 – Plan your meals for the week, even if that plan includes seven healthy frozen dinners. Make a grocery list.

Day 2 – Replace a high-calorie snack such as chips with a healthier option such as a handful of almonds or raw vegetables with fat-free ranch dip or salsa.

Day 3 – Exercise when you first wake up.

Day 4 – Adapt your favorite recipes to make just enough for you and your family.

Day 5 – Limit caloric beverages today (no regular soda pop, no sweetened tea or coffee, no juice drinks).

Day 6 – When you feel hungry, drink a glass of water or take a brief walk then assess your true level of hunger.

Day 7 – Be sure to include several servings of fruits and vegetables each day.

WEEK 36
Limit Leftovers

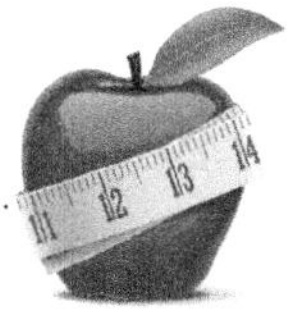

TODAY, THERE ARE so many food choices available it may be difficult to choose. Inability to limit choices may lead to overeating. Be deliberate about your food choices. When you are hungry, stop and think about what you really want to eat or what you have already planned to eat. If you don't, you may find that you've sampled your way to 200 to 300 calories without realizing it and without even having had a meal. Make a point of selecting your whole meal before you sit down to eat. Then, savor every bite. Eat slowly and truly enjoy the food.

Eat until you are satisfied, not stuffed, even if that means leaving some food on your plate or having leftovers. Most people find it difficult to waste food. Remember, the fact that the food went into your mouth rather than into the trash does not prevent poor children in third world countries from starving. If the leftovers that should have been stored away are instead eaten in a moment of weakness, they may well lead to weight gain. This in turn could lead to adult-onset diabetes or elevated cholesterol and triglyceride levels. Will a doctor visit or the cost of medication to treat the disorder cost less than those extra spoonfuls of mashed potatoes and gravy that you were afraid of wasting? The "clean plate club" mentality needs to go away.

Instead, try to be savvy when preparing meals and make just enough for a meal or be prepared to portion and freeze leftovers for another meal. The money you save by preparing less food could be donated to those in need. It may benefit you to keep the following quote from Socrates in mind, "Thou shouldst eat to live, not live to eat."

Steer clear of empty calorie, fancy coffee drinks. A 16 oz. café mocha contains about 400 calories.

Questions to Consider:

- Do you find it difficult to leave food on your plate even if you are full?
- Do you pop food into your mouth while preparing meals or while putting away leftovers?

WoW
Working on Weight Loss

Day 1 – Eat only while sitting at the table. Do not eat or drink high-calorie beverages while standing, watching TV, or working on the computer.

Day 2 – Eat only when you are hungry.

Day 3 – Allow yourself 20 minutes to finish your meals.

Day 4 – Portion food onto your plate before sitting down to eat. Do not put serving bowls on the table.

Day 5 – Do not eat any snack other than a fruit or vegetable today.

Day 6 – Eat only one serving of each food at the meal, no second helpings.

Day 7 – When storing leftovers, avoid eating any of them.

WEEK 37

Plan for the Unexpected

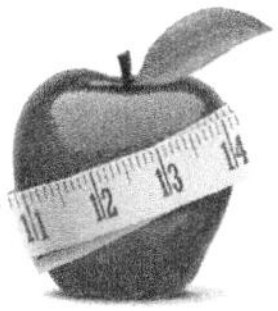

BE PREPARED. JUST as in any other scenario—being prepared pays off. How many times have you been running errands, driving from one appointment to another, or stuck in an airport and realized you were starving? Rather than wolfing down two packs of your kids "fruit" snacks, chips, or the roll of Lifesavers you found in your glove box, be prepared. Carry small bags of almonds or raisins with you. If you know you'll likely need a snack, carry fresh fruit—apples and bananas are easy to eat on the go. (One medium banana is about 100 calories; one medium apple is about 75 calories.)

What about at the office? You skipped breakfast and now the box of doughnuts in the break room is calling your name. First of all, don't skip breakfast. See Week 10 to understand why breakfast is the most important meal of the day. Second, have healthy options in your desk if possible—healthy granola, breakfast bars, or instant oatmeal. Preportioned boxes of raisins or small fruit cups are always better choices than the mini doughnuts or packaged pastry in the vending machine. You can also fix a quick dinner for that unexpected evening that brings you home later than usual. Cook some whole wheat spaghetti noodles while you thaw some frozen meatballs, to which you add prepared spaghetti sauce. Heat up a canned vegetable such as green beans or prepare frozen broccoli. Open a bag of mixed greens and dinner is ready.

To stay prepared for the unexpected, make a list of quick and easy meals and post it in the kitchen. The list may include some of the following:

- Have breakfast for dinner with whole grain waffles topped with fresh or canned fruit and your favorite eggs (boiled or scrambled whites).
- Healthy frozen dinners of your choice.
- Baked potatoes stuffed with canned chili, cottage or shredded cheese and broccoli, diced meat, salsa, and black beans. Add a lettuce salad or fruit salad for a healthy meal.
- Taco-seasoned meat over baked tortilla chips and lots of lettuce for a taco salad. Serve with a side of fruit.
- Grilled or baked chicken, instant brown rice and a frozen vegetable.
- Heat a can of black beans sprinkled with grated parmesan cheese and serve with brown rice and a serving of fruit.

- Quesadillas made with thawed, diced, frozen meatballs (or any leftover meat), shredded cheese packed between high fiber flour tortillas and grilled. Serve with salsa and low calorie sour cream and lettuce salad.

To be ready for the unexpected, keep the following items in the pantry or freezer: frozen, whole wheat buns or ready-to-bake rolls; frozen, whole grain waffles; frozen meatballs; healthy frozen dinners; frozen bags of low-fat shredded cheese (which will last for two to three months and can easily be broken apart for the amount you need without thawing the entire bag); frozen meats; frozen veggies or fruits; canned fruits and veggies; canned chili; whole grain pasta or rice; baked chips; and baking potatoes. If you are following a low-sodium diet, unprocessed foods such as fresh meats, fruits, vegetables, and grains will be lower in sodium than the convenience items that are already prepared for you.

Questions to Consider:

- Do I find myself unprepared for meals or snacks?
- Do I get so busy I forget to eat and, therefore, overindulge later?

Day 1 – Check out possible healthy snacks at the grocery store.

Day 2 – Prepare and stock healthy snacks for five days.

WoW Working on Weight Loss

Day 3 – Stock your freezer with healthy frozen dinners to use when you don't have time to cook.

Day 4 – Plan meals for a full week. Remember, some days your lunch or dinner could be leftovers, slow-cooker meals, or something as simple as a baked potato with cottage cheese and salsa.

Day 5 – Purchase groceries for the week from your carefully planned shopping list.

Day 6 – Precook any items possible, such as the meats, so only chopping, heating, etc. needs to be done the day of meal.

Day 7 – Always have whole grain cereal and milk available for breakfast.

WEEK 38

Don’t Mistake Thirst for Hunger

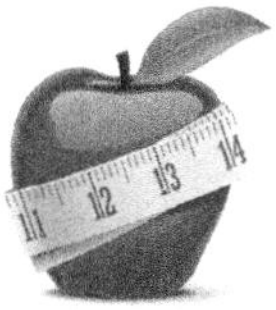

DRINK WATER BEFORE meals to curb your appetite. Limit or completely avoid high-calorie, sweetened drinks such as soda pop or other sugary beverages. Limit high-fat and sugary coffee drinks as well. These drinks contain lots of calories but have no nutritional value. Beverages such as 100 percent fruit juice or low-fat milk products contain many necessary vitamins, minerals, and phytochemicals to keep you healthy. Nutrition labels on beverages list calories for a standard eight-ounce serving, but most beverage containers have 12 to 20 ounces each. Therefore, it is important to calculate the actual calories that may be two to two-and-a-half times the listed amount.

Significant caloric intake and weight gain have recently been attributed to beverages. There are numerous sugary hot and cold drinks readily available such as soda pop, energy drinks, and coffee drinks. Some of these beverages are inexpensive to purchase, but they can be very costly to your health. High-calorie beverages create a great impact because they are typically consumed in addition to regular meals and snacks rather than in place of other calories.

There is also good reason to limit alcohol. Not only does alcohol contain a lot of calories, but the mixes further increase the number of calories in the drink. Consuming alcohol may also cause impaired judgment that leads to overeating.

Be sure to get enough fluids daily while being mindful of the calories consumed. All beverages count as a fluid (water, milk, juice, coffee, tea, etc.). You should drink enough fluids to make your urine a light, yellow color.

You may not need to gulp a sports drink during exercise unless you are sweating heavily or exercising intensely for more than an hour. If you opt for a 30-minute walk, you will likely burn 200 calories. Most sports drinks have 100 calories in a 16-ounce serving. If you drink one, then you've just swallowed 50 percent of your exercise expenditure. Water may be the best choice to keep you hydrated without defeating the purpose of your workout.

Vitamin-enhanced beverages are quite popular. Although many of these drinks are reduced-calorie or calorie-free, it may be wise to do a cost and nutrient comparison. A standard multivitamin typically contains the same nutrients plus some and likely costs less. You could afford to buy a multivitamin, fresh fruits, and vegetables for the cost of a vitamin-enhanced beverage.

When you feel like eating, stop and ask whether you are truly hungry. Perhaps you are only thirsty. Try a drink of water, a calorie-free drink, or perhaps a cup of hot tea. Then ask yourself again if you are hungry.

Questions to Consider:

- If I think I'm hungry, do I always reach for food?
- Do I have low-calorie drinks readily available throughout the day?

Day 1 – Write down everything you drink today, including water. Be sure to also record the amount consumed.

Day 2 – How much water did you drink today?

Day 3 – How many calories did you get from your beverages? Was any beverage more than 100 calories? If so, was it nutritious, such as skim milk, or just full of empty calories from sugar, like soda pop or sweetened tea?

Day 4 – Eliminate one sugary beverage (soda pop, sugared fruit drink, or energy drink) daily for one full week.

Day 5 – If you don't like water, try a carbonated version such as Pellegrino or La Croix and mix with a splash of fruit juice or fresh-squeezed lemon.

Day 6 – Put your water in a thermal cup to keep it icy cold for hours.

Day 7 – Substitute a low-calorie coffee drink for your usual latte.

WEEK 39

Celebrate Your Victories

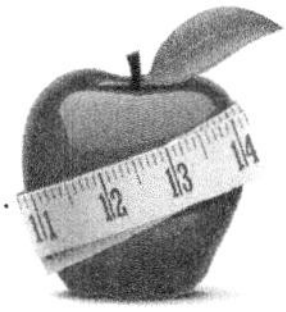

ON YOUR JOURNEY to weight loss, each day will be filled with tiny achievements. You need to recognize them. Why? Because these tiny achievements *will* accumulate. For instance, if you avoid eating one cookie (48 calories) each day, you could lose another five pounds per year. Or better yet, if you have a small, one-ounce bag of potato chips rather than finishing off half of an eight-ounce bag (608 calories) of chips, you could drop 56 pounds in a year.

Along your weight loss journey, don't compare yourself to others or seek perfection. You need to run your own race. You need to focus on your goals and accomplishments. When you do have a victory, you should celebrate it with non-food rewards. Get your nails done, purchase tickets to a local sporting event, lock the bathroom door and take a long bubble bath, go window shopping at an exclusive mall or area of town, or just enjoy a movie. If you are seeking perfection, all you'll really find is discouragement and frustration because no one is perfect. Turn your focus from food to fellowship, and you'll become a more fruitful person not only in the weight loss arena but in other areas of your life as well.

Questions to Consider:

- Do I get frustrated when I eat something I shouldn't?
- Can I find a way to celebrate that doesn't involve food?
- Do I look for achievements or for failures?

Day 1 – Write down one achievement you accomplish each day this week.

Day 2 – Ask your partner, co-worker, or friend to alert you to positive steps you have taken.

Day 3 – Look at your current weight loss (even if it's five pounds) and tell yourself you can continue your journey one step at a time.

Day 4 – Write down the behaviors you have already changed and become more determined than ever to meet your goals.

Day 5 – Recognize that losing just one pound each week will translate into 52 pounds in a year. Small achievements do add up.

Day 6 – Don't focus on food today, just enjoy your family and friends.

Day 7 – Reread the accomplishments you wrote down each day this week and celebrate them by doing something that doesn't involve food.

WEEK 40

Take a Daily Multivitamin

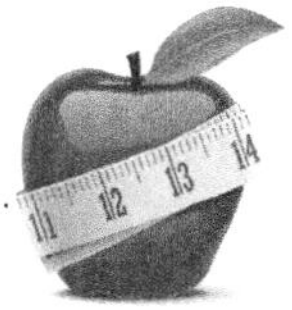

UNLIKE CARBOHYDRATES, PROTEINS, and fats, vitamins do not contain any calories, but like other nutrients, vitamins are necessary for life. If we ate a balanced diet every day, most of us would receive all the vitamins and minerals we need to function properly. Unfortunately, many people do not eat a balanced diet; therefore, taking a daily multivitamin is beneficial.

However, because a lack of certain vitamins can cause deficiency diseases such as blindness from lack of Vitamin A or rickets in children from lack of vitamin D, many people assume that "more is better" and take individual vitamin supplements. Just as a lack of intake can cause harm, taking too much can also cause harm. It may be surprising to some that even though a vitamin is essential to life, it can be harmful if taken in excess. Actually, the effects of taking almost any substance in excess can cause harm. This is the main reason why people should not self-prescribe various supplements for their health. If you don't eat properly or you typically eliminate one food group (such as meat for strict vegetarians or milk for lactose-intolerant people), taking a daily multivitamin/mineral supplement will improve your nutritional status. They can also improve your body's defenses, especially in cases when you have gastrointestinal (GI) problems.

You'll get more nutrients if you make your salads using spinach leaves or Romaine rather than iceberg lettuce. Add color and more nutrients with carrots, tomatoes, and peppers.

Inadequate vitamin/mineral intakes have been linked to chronic diseases such as heart disease, some cancers, and osteoporosis. Therefore, some physicians will recommend that their patients take a daily multivitamin. The most recent statement from the National Institutes of Health acknowledges that evidence is insufficient to recommend either for or against the use of supplements to prevent chronic diseases. Beware of marketing ploys that would have you believe you must take specific vitamins or minerals to be at your best. Taking a daily multivitamin/mineral supplement won't hurt and may help. Remember, store brands are probably just as good as nationally advertised brands and are usually less expensive because the price doesn't have to cover the cost of national advertising.

Questions to Consider:

- Do I currently take a multivitamin/mineral supplement?
- Do I currently take individual vitamin and mineral supplements?

Day 1 – Check out the labels on your nutritional supplements. The FDA does not allow companies to make claims about specific diseases unless they are supported by significant scientific evidence. (For example, the B vitamin folate protects against neural tube birth defects.)

Day 2 – To obtain information on any supplements you're taking, find consumer information from the U.S. Pharmacopeia at www.usp.org

Day 3 – Remember foods offer more than supplements including water, fiber, an abundance of phytochemicals and antioxidants, plus they stimulate the GI tract to keep it healthy.

Day 4 – Minimize destruction of essential vitamins in fruits and vegetables that have been cut by storing them in airtight wrappers and by storing juices in closed containers.

Day 5 – Minimize vitamin and nutrient losses by refrigerating your fruits and vegetables.

Day 6 – To prevent loss of nutrient content, wash fruits and vegetables before cutting.

Day 7 – Minimize nutrient losses of water-soluble vitamins (B and C) during cooking by using a microwave or steaming in a small amount of water. Add vegetables after the water has come to a boil. Also avoid high temperatures and long cooking periods.

WEEK 41

Involve Family and Friends

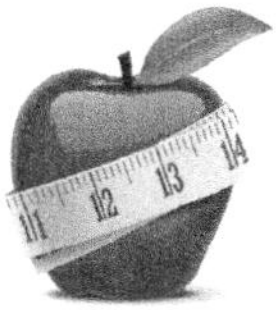

HOW AND WHY you eat is as important as what you eat. It's never too early for children to learn about healthy eating and never too late to change the habits of an adult. We all need to make healthy eating a priority. A simple key to success is eat smart and move often.

It is not what you are going through...it is what you are going to.

Serve regular, balanced family meals and snacks. Turn off televisions, video games, and computers during meals. Look for ways to spend fun, active time together. Have your family help plan the dinner menu for the week. If you have fussy children, be sure to keep adding new foods while keeping some favorite entrees or side dishes day to day. You may need to offer a new food up to 10 times before family members (especially small children) will accept it. Limit fats, sugars, and caloric drinks. Be sure the whole family participates. Ask your partner and children to each select one healthy item for purchase. Avoid purchasing unhealthy items that might tempt you later. It is much easier to stick with an eating plan if you prepare in advance.

Questions to Consider:

- Have any of my family members participated in my previous attempts to lose weight?
- Is my family involved in planning meals?

Day 1 – Use smaller plates and bowls for everyone in the family.

Day 2 – Add one new healthy food or recipe to your menu each week. Ask everyone to try it.

Day 3 – Set realistic, healthy goals for everyone.

Day 4 – Begin your meal with a salad, soup, fruit, or vegetable then enjoy the main course.

Day 5 – Pick a food item being served at dinner. Have everyone guess the portion size then measure it to see who wins.

Day 6 – Have each family member plan one meal or snack this week.

Day 7 – Have dinner out only once this week.

WEEK 42

Improve Your Mood

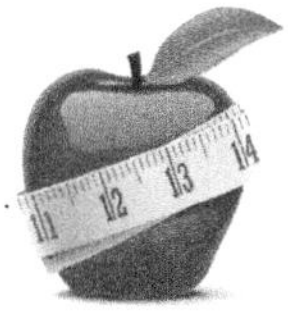

YOU PROBABLY WOULD not be surprised to learn that chocolate is the most sought-after food when people feel low. David Benton, PhD, a professor of psychology at the University of Wales, says, "Consuming chocolate hits a physiological button in the brain that triggers pleasure." Chocolate is also rich in antioxidant compounds that improve cardiovascular health by relaxing blood vessels and improving blood flow. Buy dark chocolate that is close to 60 to 70 percent cocoa. The Academy of Nutrition and Dietetics says that cravings are real, and, as long as portions are kept under control, items such as chocolate can be included in a sensible meal plan.

Carbohydrate foods (bread, pasta, rice, fruits, and veggies) have also been shown to improve mood. Eating carbohydrates during times of stress increases levels of serotonin, a stress-reducing chemical. That's why many people use carbohydrate foods as a self-medication when they feel low. However, you need to select the correct ones so that you don't add extra calories to your day's meal plan. Stay away from high-fat carbs like doughnuts, pastries, cookies, or candy. Look for whole grain breads and cereals or complex carbs like fresh fruits and vegetables. To keep your blood sugar and mood on an even keel, don't go more than four to five hours between your meals or snacks.

Population studies show lower rates of depression in societies that consume higher amounts of fish. Fish, such as tuna and salmon, is high in omega-3 fatty acids. They have been shown to promote heart health as well.

Anyone who has to have his or her morning cup of coffee to get the day started off right knows that caffeine has beneficial effects on mood. However, doses above 500 mg (about four cups) can have adverse effects. Take it easy with caffeine. With so many different coffee and energy drinks now available, it's also difficult to know exactly how much caffeine you are actually drinking. Stick with a lower amount, and you should be OK.

Questions to Consider:

- Do I always look for chocolate or a high-carbohydrate food when I'm moody?
- Can I eliminate my grouchy state by eating cookies or candy?
- Do I feel worse after eating too many goodies?

Day 1 – Go ahead and have that cup of coffee to get you going in the morning. Go easy on the cream and sugar if you add them.

Day 2 – Don't forget that tea and some soda pops also contain caffeine.

Day 3 – Purchase a bar of chocolate that's 60 percent cocoa and portion out a one- to two-ounce serving that will fit into your day's meal plan.

Day 4 – Stock up on whole grain carbohydrate foods (breads, cereals, or light popcorn) that you can eat when you need a mood lifter. As with the chocolate bar, portion them out to fit your meal plan.

Day 5 – Try to incorporate some type of fish into at least two meals per week. The fish should be grilled, broiled, or poached, not fried.

Day 6 – If you need a "mood boost" at work some days, keep one of the above mentioned foods in your desk drawer for such an occasion.

Day 7 – Time your meals or snacks to occur every four to five hours. Set your cell phone to alarm if necessary.

WEEK 43

Think Moderation, Not Deprivation

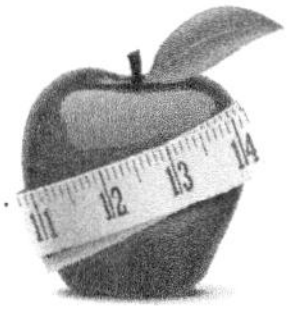

REMEMBER THE OLD phrase, "everything in moderation"? This holds true for food consumption as well. The people who are most successful at maintaining long-term weight loss are those who practice moderation rather than deprivation. With human nature being what it is, we all know that as soon as we tell ourselves we can't have something, we want it all the more. To make matters worse, whatever we decide to give up seems to haunt us on a daily basis. Tell yourself you won't eat chocolate, and, all of a sudden, chocolate is everywhere. The only thing on anyone's office desk contains chocolate; the dessert offered at the church bazaar is chocolate; the special at your usual restaurant is chocolate. The only way to solve such a dilemma is to not deprive yourself of chocolate. A small amount won't make that much difference in your daily caloric intake. Have a few M&M's,

taste that chocolate dessert at the bazaar, and split the restaurant dessert with the three other diners.

Don't worry about being perfect. Everyone has had a moment (or two or three) when they've eaten with reckless abandon. It is not surprising. Food is all around us. We cannot even go to the gas station, book store, or home improvement store without seeing a wide variety of calorie-laden drinks and snacks. If you do give into the urge to indulge, the key is to get back on track. Recognize that you overdid it this time and move on. If you don't, you will not be successful at attaining and maintaining a healthy weight and a healthy lifestyle.

Still enjoy your favorites: stuff an omelet with lean ham and veggies like broccoli, peppers, tomatoes, or onions and low fat sharp cheese.

Long-term deprivation is typically not successful, and it can be dangerous. The average adult needs about 15 percent of their daily calories from fat to keep their body functioning as it should. Many people think drastically cutting calories will help them lose weight faster. Actually, too few calories can lead to problems. It can decrease your metabolism and keep you from meeting your nutrient needs. Remember your ultimate goal is losing weight and keeping it off. If you radically restrict your food intake, your body will adjust by burning fewer and fewer calories. This is exactly the opposite of what you want to happen. Eat in moderation, and your body will continue to burn calories; exercise will also burn more calories.

Questions to Consider:

- Have my past diets deprived me of many foods I enjoy?
- Do I only think of diets as long lists of foods I should not eat?
- Can I rethink weight loss as a healthy lifestyle and not a strict diet?

Day 1 – Begin today with the statement, "I'm going to eat everything in moderation today."

Day 2 – Decide to enjoy a healthy portion of a favorite food today.

Day 3 – Look over the label of your favorite snack item and calculate the amount that will fit into your meal plan.

Day 4 – Go to a web site that calculates calories from recipes, such as http://caloriecount.about.com/cc/recipe_analysis.php. Key in your "special dessert" and see how much you can eat and still stay within your calorie allotment.

Day 5 – Look at a magazine while you wait in line at the grocery store so that you won't look at the many snacks placed there to tempt you.

Day 6 – Tell yourself, "I'm not on a diet, I'm just eating healthy!"

Day 7 – Reward yourself for staying on track.

WEEK 44

To Use or Not to Use: Sugar Substitutes

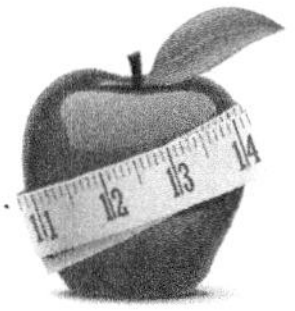

ALMOST EVERYONE LIKES something sweet; after all, the preference for sweets is inborn. In order to control their weight or prevent tooth decay, many people turn to alternative sweeteners. While unlimited intake of alternative sweeteners is not encouraged, they may be used as a substitute for sugar-laden products such as soft drinks. Bear in mind, there is no magic bullet, including sugar substitutes, for weight loss. Products other than beverages, such as yogurt, may also contain alternative sweeteners. There are various types of sweeteners available—artificial sweeteners, sugar alcohols, and natural sweeteners.

Some people have challenged the safety of using artificial sweeteners because of studies from the 1970s linking saccharin to bladder cancer in rats. (Animal studies have shown toxic effects when given in unrealistically large doses, such as the equivalent of 800 cans of diet soda daily for a lifetime.) Numerous research studies now confirm that artificial sweeteners are generally safe in limited amounts. As a result, the warning label for saccharin was dropped. Also, an article in the journal *Critical Reviews in Toxicology* reviewed over 500 studies dealing with the use of aspartame and the overall effect on health. The panel found no evidence that aspartame had negative effects on the body or mind.

Others have questioned if using artificial sweeteners can increase a person's hunger or lead to weight gain. Most randomized studies show no difference in hunger and find that people do not increase their food intake when diet soft drinks replace regular ones.

Many Americans consume 30 tsp. of added sugar per day. That's about 500 cal (more than 2 doughnuts). Cut that in half and lose 25 pounds in a year.

Artificial sweeteners are synthetic sugar substitutes but may be made from naturally occurring substances, such as herbs or even sugar itself. Their sweetening power is at least 100 times sweeter than regular sugar, so only a small amount is needed, which makes them virtually non-caloric. They typically do not raise blood sugar because they are not a carbohydrate. The FDA has established an acceptable daily intake (ADI) for each artificial sweetener. An ADI is the maximum amount that is considered safe to consume each day over the course of your lifetime. ADIs are about 100 times less than the smallest amount that might cause health concerns. The Food and Drug Administration currently has approved the use of five different artificial sweeteners: acesulfame potassium (Sunett, Sweet One); saccharin (Sweet'N Low, Sugar Twin); aspartame (NutraSweet, Equal); sucralose (Splenda), and neotame.

Sugar alcohols are another type of sugar substitute. They are carbohydrates that occur naturally in certain fruits and vegetables, but they can also be manufactured. They are found in many processed foods, replacing sugar. They are not sweeter than sugar. They do have calories but have fewer than sugar. Because they are carbohydrates, they can raise blood sugar, but not as much as sugar will because they are not completely absorbed. The FDA regulates sugar alcohols as food additives and has labeled several as generally recognized as safe (GRAS). You will find these sugar alcohols listed on ingredient labels: erythritol, isomalt, hydrogenated starch hydrolysates, lactitol, maltitol, mannitol, sorbitol, and xylitol.

Natural sweeteners are often promoted as healthier than sugar or sugar substitutes. However, these may also undergo processing and refining. They contain the same number of calories as sugar. Natural sweeteners generally recognized as safe (GRAS) by the FDA include: date sugar, maple syrup, honey, molasses, and agave nectar.

The FDA has not approved the use of whole-leaf stevia as a sweetener. Only highly refined stevia preparations (Rebaudioside A or rebiana) can be used in food products. Stevia is several hundred times sweeter than sugar. Currently, it is readily available on the market, blended with other sweeteners and sold as Truvia or PureVia.

Another sweetener that is GRAS by the FDA is tagatose. It is a low-carbohydrate sweetener similar to fructose that occurs naturally but is also manufactured from milk sugar.

There is no health benefit to consuming any type of sugar or sugar substitute. Remember that just because a food is sugar-free, does not mean it is calorie-free. The best practice is moderation when using both sugar and sugar substitutes just as you should with any other food.

Questions to Consider:

- Do I currently use artificial sweeteners?
- How much sweetener do I use on a daily basis?
- Am I replacing beverages such as milk with diet drinks? Milk provides needed protein and calcium that diet drinks do not contain.

Day 1 – What is your favorite beverage? If it is not water, take a look at the ingredients to see what is used as a sweetener.

Day 2 – Check your nutrition labels. Many foods containing artificial sweeteners still have calories and carbohydrates.

Day 3 – Keep track of the amount of artificial sweetener you place in beverages or on foods like cereal. Calculate how much sugar it would take to replace the sweeteners. Can you afford those extra calories? One teaspoon of sugar provides 16 calories.

Day 4 – If you follow a 1,600-calorie weight loss plan, you should be able to include three teaspoons of regular sugar each day without exceeding your caloric limit. According to the USDA Food

Guide, you can have the following: for a 1,800 calorie plan – 5 tsp.; for 2,000 calories – 8 tsp.; for 2,200 calories – 9 tsp.; and for 2,400 calories – 12 tsp.

Day 5 – Check out these equivalent sweetness numbers: 1 tsp. white sugar = 1 tsp. honey, 1 tsp. jam, 1½ oz. carbonated soda, or 1 Tbsp. ketchup.

Day 6 – Beware of those large soft drinks sold in convenience stores. A 40-ounce cola provides about 500 calories.

Day 7 – If you don't enjoy drinking plain water, try drinking a carbonated water mixed with a splash of 100 percent fruit juice for flavoring.

WEEK 45

Understanding Probiotics

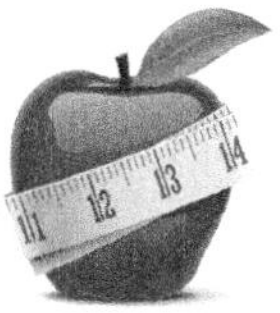

PROBIOTICS HAVE BEEN defined as live microorganisms which, when eaten in adequate amounts, have a health benefit. Probiotics help boost the immune system and stimulate digestion while replenishing the good bacteria in the intestines. The probiotic bacteria need to be alive and active. Bifidobacteria and Lactobacilli are the most commonly found probiotics added to food.

At present, dairy foods and beverages are the best products to deliver probiotics because they have a short shelf life and help neutralize stomach acid—both of which help to ensure that the probiotics are active and effective when you consume them. Some of the products that typically have probiotics include yogurt, cultured dairy products, miso, and kefir (a creamy, fermented milk product that is either plain or fruit-flavored and found in the refrigerator section of some grocery stores).

Although probiotics in food are preferred, probiotic supplements are available in various forms including freeze-dried powders, capsules, water, and liquids. To make sure these supplements remain effective, they need to be refrigerated and packaged in air-tight containers. Liquid supplements only last a few weeks. Capsules may be the best form because they usually have special coatings that protect the probiotics from being destroyed by stomach acids. As always, an individual should consult his or her physician before taking any dietary supplement. There may be food and drug interactions to consider.

Probiotics need fuel to function, and that fuel is prebiotics. Prebiotics are carbohydrates that your body cannot digest. They are found naturally in fruits and vegetables, such as bananas, asparagus, artichokes, tomatoes, onions, garlic, and in whole grains such as barley and wheat.

In addition to boosting the immune system and improving digestive health, recent studies have found that when probiotics and prebiotics are eaten, they may have positive effects on the levels of fat in your blood. Others have suggested that probiotics can be beneficial for weight loss. However, further studies are needed, and probiotics should not be used in place of any prescribed medication without first discussing the topic with your physician. Because probiotics should be consumed regularly, it is best to choose a food that is low-calorie and otherwise supports your road to health.

Questions to Consider:

- How can I incorporate probiotics and prebiotics into my daily eating?
- Does my current brand of yogurt contain active cultures?

WoW Working on Weight Loss

Day 1 – Read the label of your current yogurt container. Does it list probiotics such as *Lactobacillus* and *Bifidobacterium*?

Day 2 – Review labels of yogurt in the refrigerator section of the grocery store. Determine which ones contain active cultures and purchase these.

Day 3 – Add acidophilus milk to your cereal at breakfast.

Day 4 – Be daring—try kefir. Begin with something readily available such as kefir, low-fat smoothies.

Day 5 – Make sure you eat prebiotics such as bananas and wheat bran. Whole wheat bran flakes with sliced bananas and acidophilus milk make a great meal to start your day.

Day 6 – Eat asparagus with your dinner for a prebiotic boost.

Day 7 – If you find you are getting bored with yogurt and other dairy products, try miso to incorporate more probiotics. Additionally, keep an eye out for products on the market, such as cereals and energy bars, fortified with probiotics. Just be sure you pick a product from a trusted manufacturer in order to be sure the probiotic is a consistent strain and is potent through its shelf life.

WEEK 46

Follow the 80–20 Rule

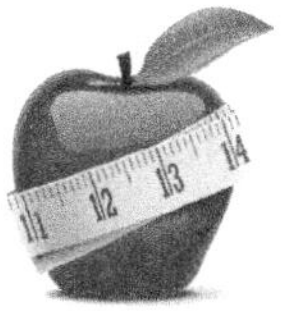

MOST PEOPLE HAVE heard of the 80-20 rule. It applies to many areas in our lives. For instance, if you run a business, you spend 80 percent of your time taking care of 20 percent of the employees who don't work out. Or, if you're a gardener, you spend 80 percent of your time taking care of the weeds that make up 20 percent of the garden. You get it, right?

Well, we can apply that same rule to weight loss. If you spend 80 percent of your time following a well-planned meal pattern, the other 20 percent will take care of itself. You have to make sure that it's only 20 percent of the time or less, not more. Let's look at the math. Three meals a day for seven days is 21 meals. Twenty percent of 21 is a little over four. For those four meals, don't make them all huge dinner meals. Perhaps a special weekend breakfast for one, two lunches on the town with a co-worker and a night out with friends or family.

Also use the 80-20 rule when you do have those special meals. Don't order an appetizer, a few cocktails, a large steak with a stuffed baked potato, and the usual high-fat, fudge brownie sundae for dessert. Keep your meal within the 80-20 parameters. Skip the appetizer or share a low-fat shrimp cocktail and have one small glass of wine. Choose an entrée that is not fried and pick steamed veggies or a baked potato with sour cream and butter on the side. Because you've done so well with dinner, go ahead and order a single slice of apple pie without the ice cream. Considering you are now at an eight on the hunger scale, divide that dessert with your dinner partner.

Make a meal from a microwave-cooked potato. Top with beans and salsa or broccoli and low-fat cheese.

If you exercise 80 percent of the time you plan to exercise, the other 20 percent will be OK. Doing some form of activity five days a week is recommended. Twenty percent of five exercise days is one day. If you need to skip your active routine once a week that's OK. The problem comes when that one day turns into two and then three. If you put off exercise one day, it becomes easier to put it off for another day, and then another day. Before you know it, exercise has become a once-a-week function. Now you have the 80-20 rule backwards. Don't let this happen to you.

Make the switch to an 80-20 lifestyle. It just might help you get through those tough times when the scale doesn't budge for a week or two. If you know you're doing what's right 80 percent of the time, the scale will eventually begin to go down again. You can stop beating yourself up over those little slip-ups. If they only happen 20 percent of the time, the other 80 percent that is on track will keep them from destroying your entire weight loss journey.

Questions to Consider:

- Do I obsess over diet plans and expect perfection from myself?
- Can I see how the 80-20 rule works in other areas of my life?

Day 1 – Allow yourself to make mistakes. When you miss your goal, get back on track right away.

Day 2 – Set a goal to prepare more home-cooked dinners this week. At the end of the week, determine if you met your goal.

Day 3 – Plan to exercise at least four days this week. Again, determine if you met your goal.

Day 4 – Check your food journal for the last week. Did you follow your meal plan 80 percent of the time?

Day 5 – If your food journal shows that you missed your mark 30 percent of the time, determine what the reason was and make plans to change that with a positive behavior.

Day 6 – If your journal shows that you missed your mark 10 percent of the time, give yourself a pat on the back.

Day 7 – Check up on your snacks today. Have you made wise choices at least 80 percent of the time?

WEEK 47

Mental Rehearsal

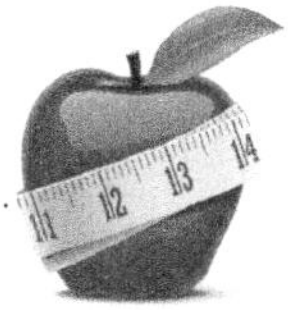

WHEN LOSING WEIGHT, we need to learn to do what Olympic and professional athletes do. It's called "mental rehearsal." Athletes have used mental rehearsal or visualization techniques for years to give themselves a competitive edge. It also appears to give them a renewed mental awareness, a heightened sense of well-being, and more confidence. Why can't we use this technique and apply it to weight loss?

Everyone knows that you can't learn a new skill without some rehearsal or practice. People who have studied these techniques tell us that we should try to imagine the "event" in great detail. Athletes rehearse over and over in their minds exactly how they will run the race, exactly how they will jump over the hurdle, or exactly how they will pitch or throw the ball. They do it so many times in their minds that it actually happens when they get to the field. We need to do it with our eating habits.

See yourself eating healthy foods. Visualize eating only small portions at the office party and enjoying the people more than the food. Before a night out for dinner, see yourself ordering a healthy entrée, see yourself enjoying half, and visualize yourself as being full. See yourself skipping dessert because you are full. Ask any good athlete, it works. And it will work for you on your journey to a healthy weight. But it takes time to develop this habit, so try some of the suggestions in the WOW section.

Questions to Consider:

- Do I see myself eating a good breakfast or just grabbing a doughnut at the office?
- Have I ever used visualization techniques in the past for sporting events or recitals?

Day 1 – See yourself eating a healthy breakfast of high-fiber cereal, low-fat or fat-free milk, and fresh fruit.

Day 2 – See yourself taking a brisk walk after lunch and enjoying the scenery.

Day 3 – See yourself in a new suit (one size smaller than before).

Day 4 – Post a picture of yourself at a lower weight on the mirror and visualize yourself at that weight again.

Day 5 – When negative images pop up, change channels to visualize a leaner, healthier you.

Day 6 – Look at your short-term goals. Check off those you have already accomplished and visualize checking off the next one.

Day 7 – Get very detailed in visualizing yourself at the next party enjoying only your favorite food in proper portions.

WEEK 48

If It Sounds Too Good To Be True...

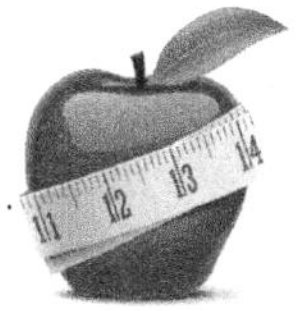

WE'VE ALL HEARD the saying, "If it sounds too good to be true, it probably is." That statement is definitely true when it come to weight loss diets. Any diet plan that promises a weight loss of 10 or more pounds per week is off-base. These plans actually give you some weight loss, but it's usually only water weight (because they dehydrate you). They are so restrictive in calories that they also reduce or eliminate required vitamins and minerals. With long-term use, these restrictive diets can be very detrimental to your overall health. In addition, any powders, potions, or beverages sold as weight loss products usually come with instructions to lower your overall calorie intake. Which is it—the powder or the lower caloric intake that brings about weight loss? You guessed it—the lower caloric intake. The diet industry takes in millions of dollars each year selling products that don't measure up to their advertised hype. The only thing getting smaller is your wallet, not your waist.

You don't need fancy diet plans that cost you a fortune or expensive exercise equipment to lose weight. Just eat less and exercise more. The problem is not many people want to hear that. They want a quick, sure-fire answer to weight loss. And the truth is, there isn't one. If there was a quick, effortless, economical, and safe weight loss plan, everyone would be doing it and there wouldn't be hundreds of diet books on the market.

Questions to Consider:

- Have I tried "crazy" diets in the past that didn't work?
- Do I want to lose weight faster than experts say I should?
- Can I be satisfied with a more reasonable weight loss plan?

Day 1 – Take a look back at previous diets you have tried. Did they promise quick weight loss? Determine to stick with only sensible eating plans and strategies found in this book.

Day 2 – Check your pantry. Have you purchased weight loss potions, drinks, or pills? Only three weight loss pills have received FDA approval. Alli is currently the only over-the-counter product that is approved. If you have other products, discard them.

Day 3 – Remind yourself about the small steps you are taking to eat healthy and exercise on most days of the week. These small steps will lead to big rewards that last.

Day 4 – Discard any diet books that promise quick weight loss or permanently eliminate any one group of food from your meal plan.

Day 5 – Remind yourself of the weight you have already lost. Even if you have reached a plateau and have not lost weight for a week or so, it's no problem. At least you didn't gain any! Once your body adjusts to the new, lower weight, you will begin to lose again.

Day 6 – Don't focus on the bathroom scale as your weight can vary as much as three pounds from day to day.

Day 7 – Check up on your most recent eating habits. Have you maintained a balance of fruits and vegetables with some starches and lean protein? Great! Keep up the good work.

WEEK 49

Myths—True or False?

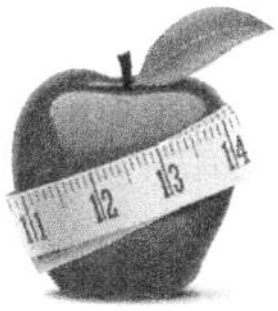

IT GOES WITHOUT saying that there are many "dieting rules" that simply are not based on scientific research. In fact, many food myths can actually add to your weight. One that you hear over and over again is that low-fat foods are lower in calories. That may be true sometimes, but to make sure, you need to read the label. You really only need to look at the calories per serving. When manufacturers take the fat out of a product, they often need to add sugar (and sometimes sodium) to make the food taste better. Some low-fat foods contain as many or more calories than their regular counterparts. Another common myth is that any fat you eat automatically becomes fat in your body. Actually, if you overeat any food (consume more calories than you burn) it will become body fat. Eating excess starches (carbs) and proteins can add extra weight just as eating excess fat can. Because fat contains twice as many calories as either carbs or protein, it's easier to overdo the fat. The fact is all people need some fat, ideally from good sources such as nuts and fish. Besides being necessary, the right kind of fat keeps you feeling full longer, so you're less likely to overeat later. Look at the following myths to help set you on the right path.

Myth: Eat the same number of calories each day.
Truth: You need to listen to your body. Our days are always different because we have more stress one day or exercise more another day. On some days you may be hungrier than others and actually need more food (fuel) for your body.

Myth: Skip a meal so you can splurge later on in the day.
Truth: If you go too long without eating, your body's metabolism slows down to conserve calories, not knowing when you will eat again. You want to keep your metabolism in high gear, not slow it down. Eat something, even if it's just an apple and an eight-ounce container of fat-free yogurt.

Myth: Potatoes and bread are both fattening, so don't eat them.
Truth: Actually starchy, high fiber vegetables and whole grain breads are good carbs that fuel your body's ability to work and think. Potatoes and bread get you in trouble when you choose to slather lots of butter or margarine on the bread and fry those potatoes. Even a healthy baked potato turns into a calorie buster when loaded with butter, sour cream, cheese, and bacon. Keep it healthy with fat-free sour cream (a measured amount) and steamed veggies such as broccoli or a nice, high-fiber, bean chili.

Myth: Women naturally gain weight after menopause.
Truth: Actually, slowing down physically is more likely the cause. Many studies have shown that older women who exercise regularly and vigorously can maintain their weight.

Myth: Diet soda is worse than the real thing.
Truth: Switching to water, green or black tea, or diluted fruit juice would be better than either regular or diet soda. Both types of soda as well as bottled cold green teas contain acids that erode tooth enamel.

Questions to Consider:

- How many of the above myths have you believed?

Day 1 – Some say muscle weighs more than fat, but a pound of either one is still a pound. The truth is muscle tissue is denser than fat tissue so it takes up less space and gives you a leaner look.

Day 2 – Drinking a glass of water before a meal to "fill you up" may be helpful. However, research shows that when water is incorporated into foods like soups, thick drinks like vegetable juices, or nectars, it tames hunger better than plain water alone.

Day 3 – If you opt for an "occasional burger and fries," it is still possible to gain weight for those who think "occasional" means every Saturday night and then some. You are better off if "occasional" means every few weeks.

Day 4 – Don't get fooled into eating one big meal each day to take off pounds. It doesn't work because it actually lowers your metabolism and tends to increase your intake when you do eat.

Day 5 – Eating fat will not automatically turn into body fat. It is only stored as fat if your caloric intake is in excess of what your body needs. Enjoy the good fats in nuts and fish to keep you feeling full longer.

Day 6 – Just as eating fat will not turn into fat; eating protein will not give you large muscles. Lean proteins, such as grilled fish or chicken, can help to keep you feeling full longer than other foods. This, in turn, can help you reduce your overall calorie intake.

Day 7 – There is some truth to chocolate cravings. Chocolate can have positive side effects. However, moderation is key. Choose to have one small (one ounce) piece of dark chocolate to satisfy your sweet cravings. Be sure to savor it while doing nothing else and then stop at one.

WEEK 50

Opt for Organic

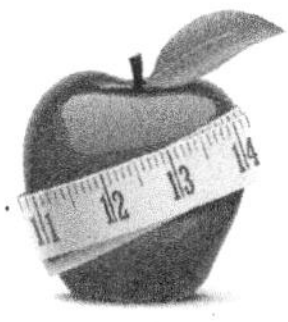

WHEN IT COMES to organic foods, the first question we need to answer is, "What *is* organic?" That question is now easier to answer thanks to the United States Department of Agriculture's National Organic program. In agriculture, *organic* means crops grown and processed according to USDA regulations defining the use of fertilizers, herbicides, insecticides, fungicides, preservatives, and other chemical ingredients.

Meat, poultry, eggs, and dairy products can be called organic if they have been raised according to the USDA regulations defining grazing conditions and the use of organic feed, hormones, and antibiotics. If a food has been irradiated, genetically engineered, or grown with fertilizer made from sewer sludge, producers cannot claim their products are organic.

Foods are certified organic when you see the green and white circle with "USDA Organic" printed inside. It means the food was produced according to strict practices that prohibit the use of synthetic flavors, colors, sweeteners, most preservatives, toxic or long-lasting pesticides, and fertilizers or methods such as genetic engineering. Producers of certified organic foods are subject to announced and unannounced inspections to make sure farming and manufacturing practices are appropriate.

When shopping for organic products, most foods are marked as such. You can also determine how fruits and vegetables are grown by reading the product code on the produce stickers. Codes for regularly grown produce contain four digits (for example, bananas have the code 4011). Codes for organic produce have five digits and begin with 9 (organic bananas have the code 94011). Codes for genetically modified produce have five digits, but begin with 8 (genetically modified bananas have the code 84011).

Whether organic foods are nutritionally superior to regular foods has been the object of recent research. For the most part, any nutrient differences reported have been within the range that normally occurs in crops. (Differences can occur with soil types, soil nutrients, and environmental conditions.) Therefore, purchasing organic (usually at a higher price) to obtain a higher level of nutrition is not wise. Purchasing organic to avoid herbicides, insecticides, fungicides, preservatives, and other chemical ingredients may be a wise move. However, don't assume that just because something is organic or good for the environment it is low in calories. You will still need to factor those calories into your daily allotment.

Some people can confuse real, certified organic foods with other terms manufacturers might use. The term "natural" on meat and poultry means that no artificial flavorings or colorings were added and that the cut of meat was not irradiated to reduce bacteria. It does not tell you anything about how the animal was raised. If any other product (cereals, canned products, etc.) uses the term "natural," it is not defined and not regulated, so, essentially, it means nothing at all.

When you see the term "free range" on chicken or eggs, it merely means the bird has had access to the outdoors. The problem is that the USDA does not regulate how much time the chicken needs to spend outdoors or on what surface. (It might be concrete). "Locally grown" is another term you often see, but exactly how far away is local? No standard exists that federal regulators can use to determine how far a food can travel and still be "local." Also remember that not all organic food is locally grown, and not all locally grown food is organic.

Questions to Consider

- Do I currently purchase organic foods?
- Do I go to farmers' markets to get fresher foods?

Day 1 – To minimize pesticide residues, select fruits and veggies that do not have holes.

Day 2 – Wash produce in running water, a veggie wash, or equal parts lemon juice and baking soda to remove residues. Rinse thoroughly.

Day 3 – Always discard the outer leaves of leafy veggies, such as cabbage and lettuce.

Day 4 – Check to see if your produce has the USDA Organic logo.

Day 5 – Foods that are the least pesticide-contaminated include onions, avocados, frozen corn, pineapples, mangoes, asparagus, frozen peas, kiwi, cabbage, eggplant, and papaya.

Day 6 – Check the codes on your produce to see if they have four or five digits.

Day 7 – Typically the produce with the most pesticide residue includes: berries, tree fruits and leafy greens. Don't eliminate them from your diet. Simply buy organic, wash well or peel.

WEEK 51
Search for Sound Information

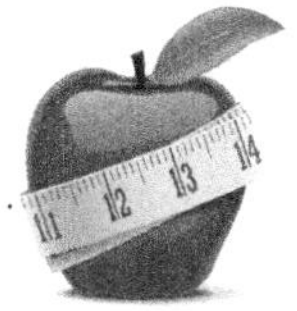

UNFORTUNATELY, IN THE world of weight loss, there are plenty of sharks promoting gimmicks that sound impressive but are not based on reliable research. Don't let yourself fall prey to them. Be cautious of what you hear on television or read in magazines and on the Internet. The most *popular* information does not necessarily mean the most *credible*. A recent study done by the American Dietetic Association found that people often pay more attention to the person providing the information than to the media that carries the message.

It is necessary to be able to recognize accurate information from misinformation. When searching for weight loss information, you will find unlimited information. Some questions you may ask yourself to determine if the information is reliable include: Is the information current? If from a website, when was the site last updated? Where is the information coming from and why? Has the information been provided by a professional with formal education in health and nutrition or a "self-proclaimed nutrition expert"? Are there references available based on research and clinical trials, or is it a personal testimonial? If the source is a website, you can learn a lot by looking at the last portion of the web address. For example:

- .gov = government websites
- .org = organization
- .edu = educational institute
- .com = commercial

Once you are confident in your ability to sort out the real from the unrealistic, you will find many tools to assist you in your quest for weight loss. There are many websites that can be referenced when determining your caloric needs and calculating BMI. Others can help you track nutritional intake throughout the day and calories burned through exercise. Still others can aid you in finding healthy recipes so that you can stick to your meal plan. If you have a smart phone, there are numerous apps available that accomplish these same tasks. These can be especially beneficial when tracking nutritional intake because you can key it in or scan the barcode as you eat rather than waiting and perhaps forgetting (or being dishonest) about what you really put into your mouth.

A few examples of helpful websites include the following:

General Nutrition Information and Weight Loss	
www.usda.gov	United States Department of Agriculture
www.nutrition.gov	United States Department of Agriculture
www.fda.gov	Food and Drug Administration
www.diabetes.org	American Diabetes Association
www.eatright.org	Academy of Nutrition and Dietetics
www.choosemyplate.gov	United States Department of Agriculture
www.cspinet.org	Center for Science in the Public Interest Nutrition Action
www.pubmed.gov	United States National Library of Medicine, National Institute of Health
www.cspinet.org/nah/	Nutrition Action Health Letter
www.mayoclinic.com	Mayo Clinic
BMR and BMI Calculator	
www.cdc.gov/healthyweight	BMI calculator – Centers for Disease Control and Prevention
www.nhlbisupport.com/bmi	BMI calculator – National Heart, Lung, and Blood Institute
www.win.niddk.nih.gov	Weight-control information network
www.healthfinder.gov	Search, "weight control," US Dept of Health & Human Services
www.nal.usda.gov/fnic	Food and Nutrition Information Center
Calorie Counter	
www.caloriecount.com	Track caloric intake
www.caloriecontrol.org	Calorie Control Council
www.nal.usda.gov/fnic/foodcomp/search/	Calorie content of foods
www.calorieking.com	Track food intake, membership fee $
www.weightwatchers.com	Track food intake, membership fee $
Exercise/Activity	
www.nutristrategy.com/activitylist4.htm	List of calories burned during exercise
www.shapeup.org	10,000 step program, Shape Up America!

Recipe Sites
www.allrecipes.com www.cookinglight.com http://caloriecount.about.com/cc/recipe_analysis.php – Recipe calculator

Applications for Smart Phones

Available apps vary based upon the type of phone you have. However, be aware that the availability of free helpful apps continues to grow.

Questions to Consider:

- Have I been using reliable resources for my weight loss information?
- Do I jump at every quick weight loss idea in print?

Day 1 – Flip through a magazine at the newsstand to see if it contains any reliable nutrition and weight loss information.

WoW Working on Weight Loss

Day 2 – Check out one of the suggested websites for new information.

Day 3 – Keep a food diary/log online, on paper, or on a smart phone app.

Day 4 – Plan meals in advance using cookbooks, magazines, or websites that give nutrition information for each recipe. If there is no nutrition information available, plug the recipe into the online recipe calculator to see how healthy it is.

Day 5 – Go to www.eatright.org and look up "popular diet reviews" to see if you are able to identify reliable nutrition advice.

Day 6 – Focus on the tips you've learned in this book and stick with those that "work" for you.

Day 7 – Pat yourself on the back for being a savvy consumer of weight loss information.

WEEK 52
Keep Your Momentum

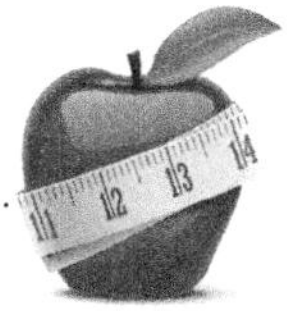

OK, SO YOU'VE been gradually dropping one to two pounds each week for some time now. Then pow! It happens. Some special occasion comes up—say a vacation—and instead of losing a pound that week you gain three or four. Whatever you do, don't stop and give up. It's not a matter of failing; it's a matter of getting up again. To give you some incentive, think back on other victories you've achieved. Think of other instances where you went wrong but didn't give up and eventually reached your goal. Hey, no one is perfect! We all slip up. Forgive yourself and move on.

Just so that you don't think you're the only one having trouble on this journey, look at data from the *National Weight Control Registry*. It includes more than 4,000 people who have lost at least

30 pounds and kept it off for one year. The average weight lost is 66 pounds for a total of five and a half years. To make it even better, 90 percent of registry members had previously tried and failed to lose weight. The majority of members ate three meals and two snacks each day, ate healthier foods in smaller amounts, and exercised regularly. They also decreased consumption of junk foods and lost weight over a longer period of time, i.e. no quick fixes. The registry members say that it takes less effort to maintain their new weight as time passes. That's positive because if the members could keep the weight off for one year, their chances of continuing to keep it off go up.

Once you've lost weight, you still need to be aware of portion sizes. You should be able to eat more when you are maintaining your weight, but not as much as you might think. Most people can only spare an additional 150 to 250 calories each day. If you order an eight-piece chicken nugget portion instead of the child's size four-piece portion, you've already added 170 extra calories. Dividing the calories between your meals is a better option and gives you 50 to 75 calories per meal. Some healthy yet satisfying additions might include one tablespoon of sunflower seeds (50 calories) to your luncheon salad; two tablespoons of grated parmesan cheese (50 calories) to your pasta for dinner; or one hard boiled or poached egg (75 calories) added to your whole wheat toast and juice for breakfast.

Questions to Consider:

- Have I set myself up to keep moving in the right direction despite mishaps?
- Do I have a list of accomplishments I can review to give me a fresh perspective?

Day 1 – Make a list of accomplishments you've achieved in the past and enjoy your victories.

WoW Working on Weight Loss

Day 2 – Do what registry members do and consume three meals and two snacks each day.

Day 3 – To get in a little more exercise, walk around the mall before heading to the first store.

Day 4 – Don't pay for gas at the pump. Always walk to the convenience store to pay and while you're at it, walk around the perimeter of the store first. Those few extra steps will eventually add up.

Day 5 – Look at the weight you have already lost and make five positive statements about your accomplishments during the day. (How about, "I'll continue to eat mostly complex carbohydrates and healthy fats.")

Day 6 – Tell your body, "I will take care of you today." Such a positive mantra can make every day a good one.

Day 7 – Recheck your pantry for any "junk" foods that have found their way back into your house. Either toss them or take them to the office to share.

APPENDICES

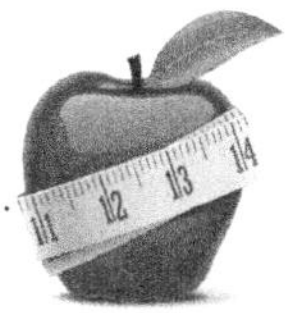

APPENDIX A: CALORIE/ACTIVITY TABLES

MOST CALORIE/ACTIVITY TABLES give you information for a 150-pound person doing an activity for 30 minutes. However, most people losing weight are not 150 pounds and are often not active for 30 minutes. Using this information to calculate how many calories you will burn at 233 pounds doing the activity for 15 minutes takes a degree in math. The table below provides an easier method for determining how many calories a person will burn for a given activity.

For example, a person weighing 256 pounds who vacuums for 35 minutes can see that he or she will burn .030 calories per pound per minute. Multiply .030 times 256 pounds times 35 minutes. It only takes a few seconds with a calculator, and you have your answer of 268.8 calories. As you lose weight, the number of calories you burn for each activity will decrease because the number of pounds you weigh will decrease. It would be best to redo the math for every 10 to 15 pounds you lose.

CALORIES BURNED DURING EXERCISE			
Activity	**kcal/lb/min**	**Activity**	**kcal/lb/min**
Aerobics (g)	.045	**Auto repair**	.022
Aerobics, high impact	.053	**Basketball (g)**	.060
Bowling	.022	**Basketball (v)**	.097
Dance(v)	.062	**Carpentry (g)**	.026
Child Care	.022	**Cleaning House (g)**	.026
Coaching	.030	**Cooking**	.019
Handball	.078	**Darts**	.019
Golf (carry clubs)	.045	**Golf (pull clubs)**	.038
Golf (power cart)	.026	**Fishing (boat)**	.019
Fishing (stand)	.026	**Fishing (stream)**	.045
Football (g)	.060	**Frisbee (g)**	.022
Gardening	.045	**Hiking (cc)**	.045
Horse Grooming	.045	**Horse Riding (g)**	.030
Kickball	.053	**Mow Lawn (g)**	.042
Riding mower	.019	**Raking Lawn**	.030
Racquetball (g)	.053	**Rope Jump (g)**	.075
Shovel Snow	.045	**Snow Ski (g)**	.045
Ski, Cross Country	.060	**Skating, ice(g)**	.053
Roller Skating	.053	**Skiing water**	.045
Rowing, stationary	.064	**Rowing (v)**	.097
Snorkeling	.038	**Snowmobiling**	.026
Stair/Treadmill (g)	.045	**Sweeping**	.030
Studying	.011	**Soccer (v)**	.097
Table Tennis	.030	**Volleyball (g)**	.022
Tennis (beginner)	.032	**Tennis, doubles**	.045
Volleyball (g)	.022	**Vacuuming**	.030

Bicycling		Running	
13 mph (g)	.045	5 mph	.061
15 mph	.049	6 mph	.074
17 mph	.057	7.5 mph	.094
19 mph (v)	.076	9 mph	103
21 mph	.090	10 mph	.114
23 mph	.109	11 mph	.131
25 mph	.139		
Walking (brisk pace)		3.5 mph	.035
Swimming		**Wii Games**	
20 yd/min	.032	bowling	.021
45 yd/min	.058	boxing	.021
50 yd/min	.070	tennis	.022

(g=general)
(v = vigorous)

APPENDIX B: BMI CHART

BMI	19	20	21	22	23	24	25	26	27	28	29	30	31	31	33	34	35
Height	Weight in Pounds																
4′10″	91	96	100	105	110	115	119	124	129	134	138	143	148	153	158	162	167
4′11″	94	99	104	109	114	119	124	128	133	138	143	148	153	158	163	168	173
5′	97	102	107	112	118	123	128	133	138	143	148	153	158	163	158	174	179
5′1″	100	106	111	116	122	127	132	137	143	148	153	158	164	169	175	180	185
5′2″	104	109	115	120	126	131	136	142	147	153	158	164	169	175	180	186	191
5′3″	107	113	118	124	130	135	141	146	152	158	163	169	175	180	186	191	197
5′4″	110	116	122	128	134	140	145	151	157	163	169	174	180	186	192	197	204
5′5″	114	120	126	132	138	144	150	156	162	168	174	180	186	192	198	204	210
5′6″	118	124	130	136	142	148	155	161	167	173	179	186	192	198	204	210	216
5′7″	121	127	134	140	146	153	159	166	172	178	185	191	198	204	211	217	223
5′8″	125	131	138	144	151	158	164	171	177	184	190	197	203	210	216	223	230
5′9″	128	135	142	149	155	162	169	176	182	189	196	203	209	216	223	230	236
5′10″	132	139	146	153	160	167	174	181	188	195	202	209	216	222	229	236	243
5′11″	136	143	150	157	165	172	179	186	193	200	208	215	222	229	236	243	250
6′	140	147	154	162	169	177	184	191	199	206	213	221	228	235	242	250	258
6′1″	144	151	159	166	174	182	189	197	204	212	219	227	235	242	250	257	265
6′2″	148	155	163	171	179	186	194	202	210	218	225	233	241	249	256	264	272
6′3″	152	160	168	176	184	192	200	208	216	224	232	240	248	256	264	272	279

APPENDIX C: UNDERSTANDING FOOD LABELS

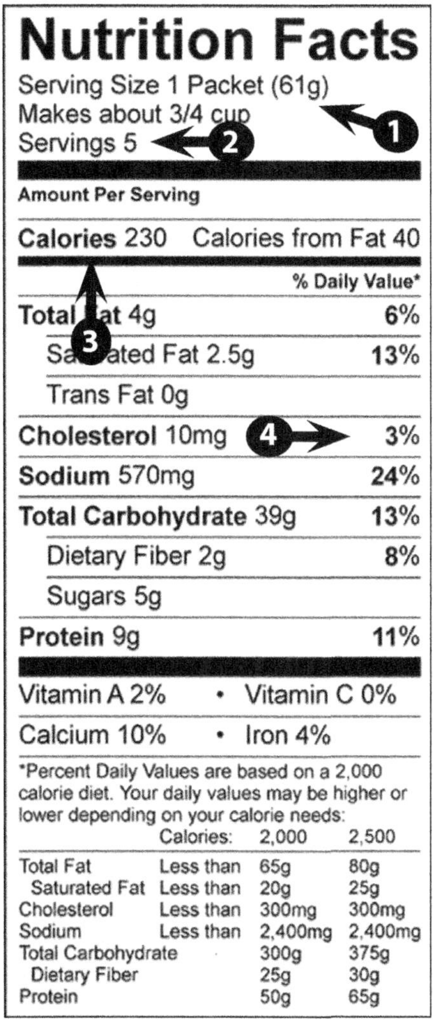

Sample label for macaroni and cheese

Key items to focus on when reading labels:

1. Serving Size: This is the portion that provides the nutrients listed on the label. You must be sure you are consuming the portion as listed or adjust nutrients accordingly.

2. Serving per Container: Don't assume that the whole container is one serving.

3. Calories per Serving: Be sure you are limiting yourself to only one serving or increasing the total calories if eating more than one serving.

4. Note that the **Percent Daily Values** are based on a 2,000 calorie diet.

APPENDIX D: HUNGER SCALE

1	You are ravenous, may be physically weak
2	You are famished, perhaps have a headache
3	Your stomach is empty and may growl
4	You are not really hungry but could nibble
5	You feel fairly satisfied
6	You feel satisfied, not hungry but not full or stuffed
7	You feel satisfied but still have room for more
8	Now you are full
9	You are now so full your clothes are tight
10	You are now stuffed and may even experience reflux

APPENDIX E: SEVENTY THINGS TO DO RATHER THAN EAT

Things to Do Inside

- Balance your checkbook. (Stand at kitchen counter to do so.)
- Wipe grimy handprints from refrigerator, stove, dishwasher, and cabinet doors.
- Toss spoiled produce from fridge's veggie bin and wash the bin in the sink.
- Clean off one shelf in fridge and wipe down all jars and bottles.
- Wipe off all spice and herb containers and reorganize them.
- Remove everything from the top of the fridge; clean items and the top.
- Quick mop your small kitchen floor. (Big kitchen? Do the dirtiest half.)
- Change the linens on one bed.
- Refold clothes in a messy drawer.
- Untangle and organize jewelry on a dresser top or in a jewelry box.
- Tidy up your closet one section at a time. (Try two- to three-foot sections.)
- Put unused clothes from closet in bags (mark "donate," "consignment," etc.) and place by front door to deliver ASAP.
- Remove everything from a small closet floor and vacuum; organize as you replace.

- Refresh one pair of sneakers by scrubbing off scratches.
- Clean off the vanity and sink in one bathroom.
- Clean off the mirror in one bathroom.
- Clean the floor in one small bathroom.
- Remove items from one or two medicine cabinet shelves, toss those outdated, and organize as you replace.
- Tidy up a small, under-sink cabinet or do half of a large one.
- Divide laundry and put a load in the washer.
- Hand wash one or two small laundry items and hang to dry.
- Iron one shirt or other piece of clothing.
- Clean the door handles and faceplates of light switches in one or two rooms.
- Empty all trash containers into one large bag and place by trash.
- Gather all old newspapers and magazines for recycling or donation.
- Do ten regular or modified pushups.
- Wipe down one good piece of wood furniture with lemon oil.
- Dust corners of rooms for cobwebs.
- Dust air vents.
- Leaf through old magazines for pages you want to keep.
- Organize your purse or briefcase.
- Wipe down the baseboards in one room.

- Take down sheer curtains and wash. (If sheer, they can go back up damp.)
- Vacuum curtains and valances in one room.
- Dust lampshades in several rooms.
- Call a best friend.
- Clean your makeup brushes.
- Determine your outfits to wear to work next week.
- Clean the top of blades to a ceiling fan.
- Clean four or five picture frames or mirrors.
- Sort through a pile of old mail.
- Clean out the microwave oven.
- Drink a glass of water.
- Vacuum two large rooms or a room and a hall.
- Read a good book.

Things to Do Outside

- Pull weeds in one section of your garden.
- Walk the dog.
- Trim the hedges on one side of your house.
- Enjoy a calorie free beverage on the back porch.
- Go for a walk with your kids.
- Wash your car or truck.
- Vacuum out the car.

- Polish your rims.
- Play ball with your child or dog.
- Go for a bike ride.
- Organize your workbench.
- Clean your outdoor grill.
- Walk around the park.
- Mow the lawn.
- Sweep off the front porch and/or sidewalk.
- Clean the windows.
- Pick some flowers for a vase.

Things to Do At The Office

- Clean out your inbox.
- Organize your desk drawers.
- Rather than phone a coworker—walk to their desk.
- Answer e-mails.
- Clean off the top of your desk.
- Take the long way (to and from) lunch.
- Chew a piece of gum.
- Walk to get a cup of unsweetened hot tea.

APPENDIX F: HEALTHY SNACK IDEAS

Sweet Tooth Snacks	
Under 50 Calories	
½ medium apple baked and topped with 1 Tbsp. low-fat yogurt sprinkled with cinnamon (45)	
½ small banana (Freeze it for a special cool treat.) (45)	
4 oz. unsweetened applesauce sprinkled with cinnamon (49)	
1 serving sugar-free gelatin with 3 Tbsp. light whipped topping (40)	
½ cup strawberries with 2½ Tbsp. nonfat yogurt (47)	
1 miniature box of raisins (45)	2 sugar-free ice pops (30)
1 sugar-free fudge ice pop (35)	12 cherries (48)
1 Miniature Reese's Peanut Butter Cup (44)	Miniature Kit Kat bar (42)
Mini York Peppermint Pattie (47)	2 Starbursts (40)
1 Fig Newton cookie (50)	1 vanilla sandwich cookie (48)
1 pkt. diet hot cocoa (25-50)	1/3 oz. of dark chocolate (50)
¼ cup (20) mini marshmallows (45)	15 semi-sweet chocolate chips (40)
Between 60 and 100 Calories	
½ cup low-fat chocolate milk (75)	1 gelatin snack pack (70)
4 large marshmallows (92)	20 Reese's pieces (80)
20 chocolate-covered raisins (80)	3 chocolate kisses (75)
4 mini Tootsie Rolls (95)	1 Oreo Double Stuff cookie (70)

Crunchy Snacks	
Under 50 Calories	
1 pretzel rod (37)	1 kosher dill pickle (10)
1½ cups sugar snap peas (40)	1 Tbsp. dry roasted sunflower seeds (47)
½ small apple w/ 1 tsp. peanut butter (46)	2 pieces beef jerky (50)
1 brown rice cake w/ 1 Tbsp. sugar free jam (44)	½ c. raw broccoli (15)
1/2 cup carrots w/ 1 Tbsp. light ranch dressing (45)	2 celery stalks (13)
2 cups of light butter popcorn (50)	
Between 60 and 100 Calories	
1/2 cup Chex mix/traditional (98)	20 mini cheese crackers (100)
1/4 cup of walnut pieces (98)	Any 100-calorie package chips (100)
1 Kudos granola bar fruit/nuts (90)	11 Sun Chips (100)
1 whole graham cracker (70)	½ cup pickled beets (74)

More Snacks	
Under 50 Calories	
1 large tomato sliced & topped w/ 1 Tbsp. parmesan cheese then broiled (44)	
½ cup plain fat-free yogurt sprinkled w/ 1 tsp. sunflower seeds (46)	
1.3 oz. water-packed tuna w/ 1 tsp. Dijon mustard (48)	
½ cup melon w/ 2 Tbsp. 1% cottage cheese (47)	
½ small grapefruit (32)	6 oz. vegetable juice (39)
½ cup cauliflower (13)	12 grape tomatoes (25)
½ cup blueberries (42)	4 melba toast crackers (50)
2 Tbsp. hummus (50)	¼ cup salsa (20)
Between 60 and 100 Calories	
¼ cup dried peaches or apricots (100)	½ cup low-fat vanilla yogurt (100)
12 almonds (80)	1 oz. mozzarella cheese (72)
½ cup low-fat cottage cheese (90)	2 oz. salmon (90)
2 oz. water packed tuna (66)	1 egg (75)

References and Further Reading

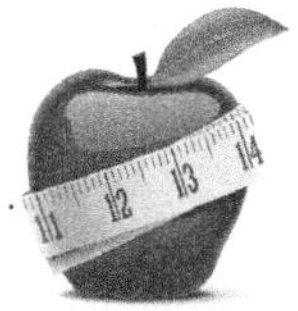

Bellisle, F. and Drewnowski, A., Intense sweeteners, energy intake and the control of body weight, *European Journal of Clinical Nutrition* 61 (2007): 691-700.

B.M. Davy and coauthors. Water consumption reduces energy intake at a breakfast meal in obese older adults, *Journal of the American Dietetic Association* 108(2008): 1236-1239.

Behavioral Treatment of Obesity. *American Journal of Clinical Nutrition, 82* (2005): 230S-235S.

Committee on Dietary Reference Intakes, *Dietary Reference Intakes for Energy, Carbohydrate, Fiber, Fat, Fatty Acids, Cholesterol, Protein, and Amino Acids* (Washington, D.C.: National Academies Press, 2005).

Comparison of Atkins, Ornish, Weight Watchers, and Zone Diets for Weight Loss and Heart Disease Reduction. *Journal of the American Medical Association, 293* (2005): (1) 43-53.

Despres, J. (2008). Abdominal obesity and the metabolic syndrome: Contribution to global cardiometabolic risk. *Arteriosclerosis, Thrombosis, and Vascular Biology*, 1039-1049.

Doran, George T. There's a S.M.A.R.T. way to write management's goals and objectives. *Management Review*, 70(11)(1981).

Dubnov-Raz G, Berry EM. Dietary approaches to obesity. Mt Sinai J Med. 2010. Sep-Oct; 77(5):488-98. PubMed PMID: 20960551.

E.L. Van Walleghen and coauthors. Pre-meal water consumption reduces meal energy intake in older but not younger subjects, *Obesity* 15 (2007): 93-99.

Farshchi, H.R., Taylor, M.A., Macdonald, I.A. Beneficial metabolic effects of regular meal frequency on dietary thermogenesis, insulin sensitivity, and fasting lipid profiles in healthy obese women. *American Journal of Clinical Nutrition* 81(2005):(1) 16-24.

Frankenfield DC, et al. Comparison of Predictive Equations for Resting Metabolic Rate in Healthy Nonobese and Obese Adults: A Systematic Review. J Am Diet Assoc. 2005;105:775-789

G.C. Major and coauthors, Clinical significance of adaptive thermogenesis, *International Journal of Obesity* 31 (2007): 204-212.

Guthrie, H. Selection and quantification of typical food portions by young adults. Journal of the American Dietetic Association. 84(1984): (12)1440-1444.

J.E. Flood and B.J. Rolls, Soup preloads in a variety of forms reduce meal intake, Appetite 49 (2007): 626-634.

J.M. Poothullil, Recognition of oral sensory satisfaction and regulation of the volume of intake in humans, *Nutritional Neuroscience* 8(2005): 245-250.

Katcher, H.I. et al., *American Journal of Clinical Nutrition* 2008 Jan; 87 (1): 79-90.

Long Term Weight Maintenance. (2005). *American Journal of Clinical Nutrition , 82* (2005): 222S-225S.

Mifflin MD, St. Jeor ST, Hill LA, Scott BJ, Daughterty SA, Koh YO. A new predictive equation for resting energy expenditure in healthy individuals. *Am J Clin Nutr.* 1990; 51:241-247.

M.L. Slattery and coauthors, Plant foods, fiber, and rectal cancer, *American Journal of Clinical Nutrition* 79 (2004): 274-281.

National Institutes of Health Obesity Education Initiative. 2000.

Patel S.R. et al., Association between reduced sleep and weight gain in women. *American Journal of Epidemiology* 2006 Nov 15; 164(10):947-954.

Pereira, D. and Gibson, G., Effects of Consumption of Probiotics and Prebiotics on Serum Lipid Levels in Humans, Critical Reviews in Biochemistry and Molecular Biology, 37 (4): 259-281 (2002).

P. Monsivais, M. M. Perrigue, and A. Drewnowski, Sugars and satiety; Does the type of sweetener make a difference? *American Journal of Clinical Nutrition* 86 (2007): 116-123.

R.N. Close and D.A. Schoeller, The financial reality of overeating. *Journal of the American College of Nutrition , 25(2006):* 203-209.

Rolls, B.J., Morris, E.L. and Roe, L.S. Portion size of food affects energy intake in normal-weight and overweight men and women. *American Journal of Clinical Nutrition*, 76(2002):1207-1213.

Rolls, B.J., Roe, L.S. and Meengs, J.S. Larger portion sizes lead to sustained increase in energy intake over two days. *Journal of the American Dietetic Association*, 106(2006):543-549.

Rolls, B.J., Roe, L.S. and Meengs, J.S. Reductions in portion size and energy density of foods are additive and lead to sustained decreases in energy intake over two days. *American Journal of Clinical Nutrition*, 83(2006):11-17.

Rolls, B.J., Roe, L.S. and Meengs, J.S. Salad and satiety: energy density and portion size of a first course salad affect energy intake at lunch. *Journal of the American Dietetic Association*, 104(2004):1570-1576.

Schwartz, J and Byrd-Bredbenner, C. Portion Distortion: Typical Portion Sizes Selected by Young Adults. *Journal of the American Dietetic Association*. 106(9) (2006): 1412-1418.

S. Liu and coauthors, Relation between changes in intakes of dietary fiber and grain products and changes in weight and development of obesity among middle-aged women, *American Journal of Clinical Nutrition* 78 (2003): 920-927.

The National Weight Control Registry (NWCR), established in 1994 by Rena Wing, Ph.D. from Brown Medical School, and James O. Hill, Ph.D. from the University of Colorado.

Vander Wall, J.S. et at., International Journal of Obesity 2008 Oct:32 (10): 1545-1551.

U.S. Food and Drug Administration, U.S. Department of Health and Human Services.

Wansink, B., van Ittersum, K., and J.E. Painter, Ice cream illusions bowls, spoons, and self-served portion sizes, *American Journal of Preventive Medicine* 31(2006): 240-243.

Zernel, M.B. et al., *International Journal of Obesity* 2005 Apr: 29(4): 391-397.

U.S. Department of Agriculture, Agricultural Research Service. USDA National Nutrient Database for Standard Reference, Release 21. 2008. Available at: http://www.nal.usda.gov/fnic/foodcomp/search/ Accessed 11/7/08.

Acknowledgements

Linda and Kim would both like to thank Marie Kamp, MS, RD (Dietetic Internship Director from Penn State University) for her expert review of this book.

Linda thanks her husband Dr. David Owens for his patience and support. She also thanks her son, Jason, and daughter, Shannon, for reviewing the book and offering suggestions about appealing to the general population. Linda's sisters also reviewed the book with suggestions on additional topics to include. Linda's sister-in-law, Helen Reneau, was of great value with her editing expertise.

Kim thanks her husband for his support during the writing of the book. She also thanks her children for selflessly sharing of their Mom-time so she could work with Linda on the book. Kim's mother and sister are also appreciated as they offered common sense critiques that proved valuable.

Author Information

Linda Owens has seen many clients struggle with weight loss over her 20 years of experience in the field of nutrition. Linda has a bachelor's and a master's degree and currently teaches nutrition at Oral Roberts University in Tulsa, Oklahoma. She has also designed and taught her own successful weight management program.

Kim Alp has participated with clients during their quest for successful weight loss in clinical settings. She holds both a bachelor's and a master's degree and has over 20 years of experience as a registered dietitian. Kim continues to practice as a registered and licensed dietitian in Tulsa, Oklahoma.

Many people have little or no success with weight loss because they try to make a fixed diet plan fit their individual situation. This book is written to incorporate small behavior and lifestyle changes that anyone can follow. It is well researched with scientific data supporting the strategies designed to lead to healthy outcomes and weight loss for the reader. Whereas we believe a one-on-one session with a dietitian is ideal, it is not always practical. Therefore, we chose to develop this book which uses small weekly sections to give individuals the tools they need for long term weight management.

Printed in Dunstable, United Kingdom

91223990R00143